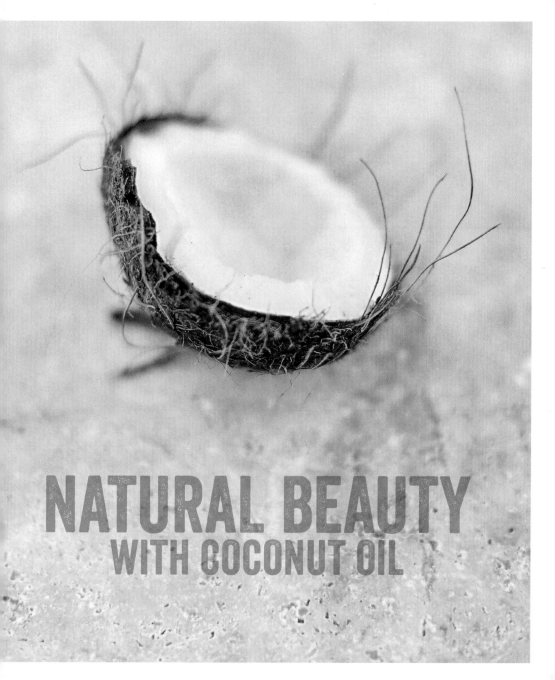

NATURAL BEAUTY
WITH COCONUT OIL

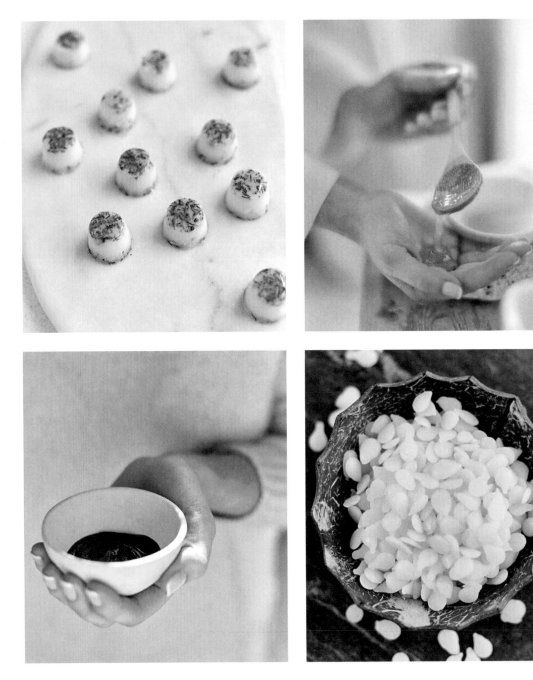

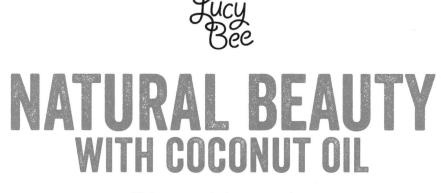

Lucy Bee

NATURAL BEAUTY
WITH COCONUT OIL

50 homemade beauty recipes
using nature's perfect ingredient

Photography by David Loftus

quadrille

PUBLISHING DIRECTOR Sarah Lavelle
COMMISSIONING EDITOR Lisa Pendreigh
PROJECT EDITOR Amy Christian
COPY EDITOR Sally Somers
BEAUTY CONSULTANT Fiona Embleton
CREATIVE DIRECTOR Helen Lewis
SENIOR DESIGNER Katherine Keeble
PHOTOGRAPHER David Loftus
RECIPE STYLIST Poppy Mahon
PROPS STYLIST Jo Harris
HAIR AND MAKE-UP Maria Comparetto
PRODUCTION DIRECTOR Vincent Smith
PRODUCTION CONTROLLER Emily Noto

With thanks to The Linen Works for loaning items
for photography.

First published in 2016 by
Quadrille Publishing Limited
Pentagon House
52–54 Southwark Street
London SE1 1UN
www.quadrille.co.uk
www.quadrille.com

Quadrille is an imprint of Hardie Grant
www.hardiegrant.com.au

Reprinted in 2016
10 9 8 7 6 5 4 3 2

Cataloguing in Publication Data:
a catalogue record for this book
is available from the British Library.

ISBN: 978 1 84949 894 4

Printed in China

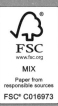

FSC
www.fsc.org
MIX
Paper from
responsible sources
FSC® C016973

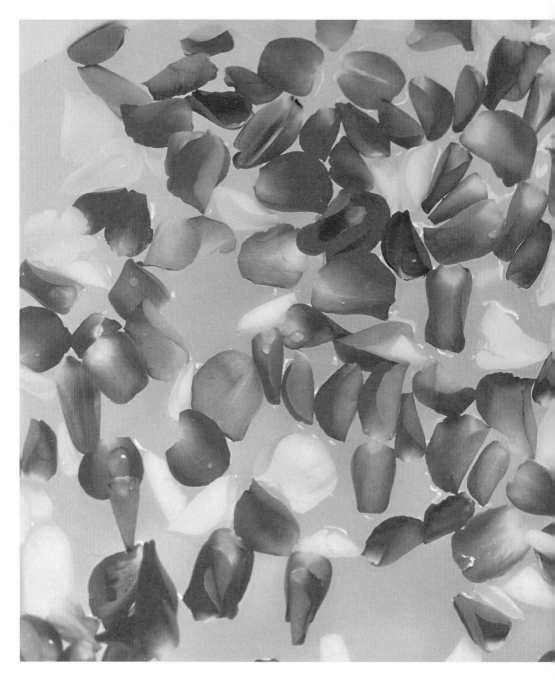

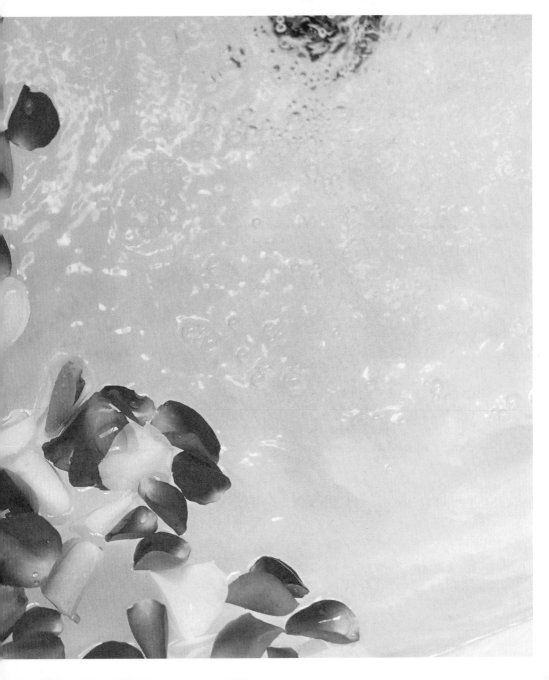

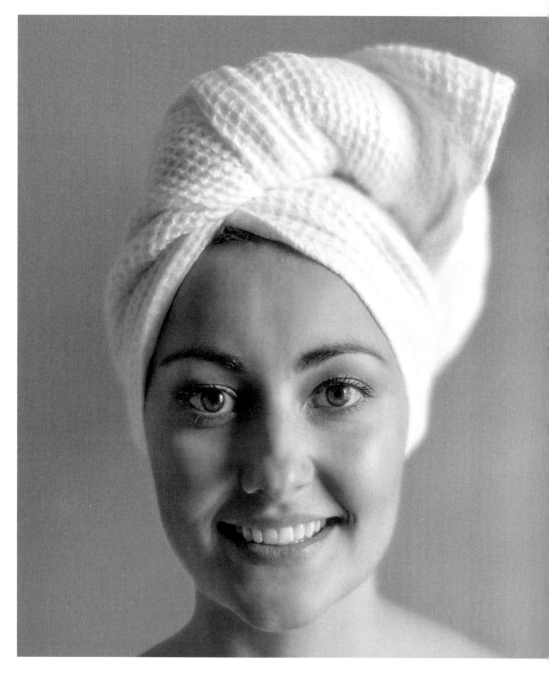

INTRODUCTION

Coconut oil is known for its versatility but can you actually believe that something you cook your roast potatoes in can be applied to your face to remove the most stubborn, waterproof mascaras? I couldn't quite believe it either when I first discovered all the ways you could use coconut oil, from a shaving cream and make-up remover to a hair mask and even as a tattoo healer. I know, sounds crazy, huh?! Well, it's true and you'll be amazed at how well it works!

That's why, as a CIBTAC qualified beauty therapist, I wanted to share my tips and ideas for natural beauty and to show you how easy it is to make your own beauty products, getting the most out of your Lucy Bee jar and other products in the range.

If you haven't heard of Lucy Bee as a brand, let me explain who we are. Lucy Bee is a family-run business: my dad is the businessman behind the scenes and I started off by running the social media side of things, which has grown into a much bigger role. Our ethos is all about using ingredients that are organic, natural, raw, and as close to nature as possible. We are also proud to be Fair Trade, which is something that we feel very strongly about.

This brings me on to what we are best known for: our coconut oil. As a family we were introduced to coconut oil and Bruce Fife's book, *The Coconut Oil Miracle*, in 2007, by a friend from Hong Kong. We soon realized what an amazing product this was for both cooking and beauty and wanted

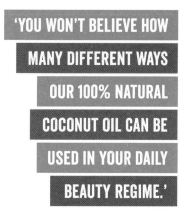

'YOU WON'T BELIEVE HOW MANY DIFFERENT WAYS OUR 100% NATURAL COCONUT OIL CAN BE USED IN YOUR DAILY BEAUTY REGIME.'

to share all that we'd learnt about it. We now have a whole range of natural products – cacao, maca, lucuma, turmeric, Epsom salts, Dead Sea salt, Himalayan salt, and cinnamon. I love the fact that most things in our Lucy Bee range work as both cooking and beauty products, since these are the two things I am most passionate about. So what makes coconut oil a great beauty product? Well, it's made up of approximately 48% lauric acid (and one of the only other places you'll find this is in breast milk). Lauric acid is full of health-boosting and skin-loving properties because it is antibacterial, antiviral, and antifungal. Coconut oil is also high in vitamin E, which is highly beneficial to the skin as well.

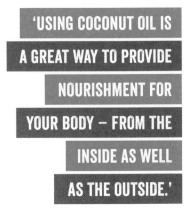

'USING COCONUT OIL IS A GREAT WAY TO PROVIDE NOURISHMENT FOR YOUR BODY – FROM THE INSIDE AS WELL AS THE OUTSIDE.'

The skin is the biggest organ in your body and it needs a lot of love, so it makes sense to care for it with natural, skin-friendly products. Just as we look at the foods that we're eating, so we should look at how our beauty products are made – and what better way to do this than to make them yourself?

I hope you enjoy the different recipes in this book and make sure you take time out of this crazy, busy life to pamper and look after yourself, both inside and out. Use this book for those times when you could just do with a helping hand to feeling your best again, or to indulge in your own, at-home, mini spa break!

Love,

Lucy Bee x

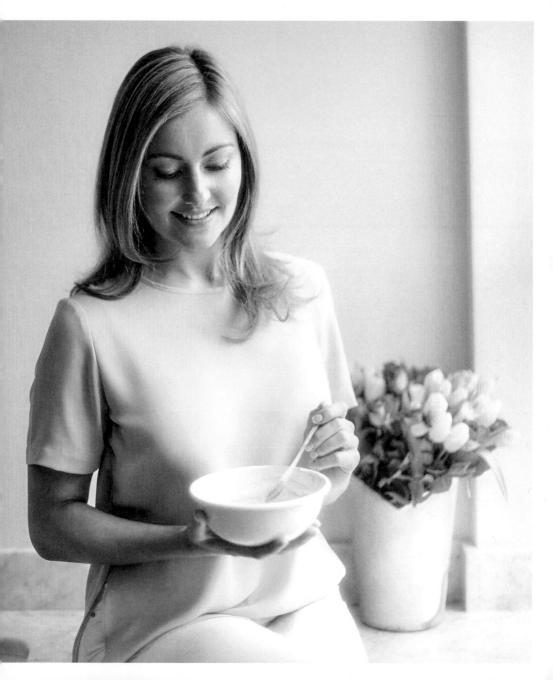

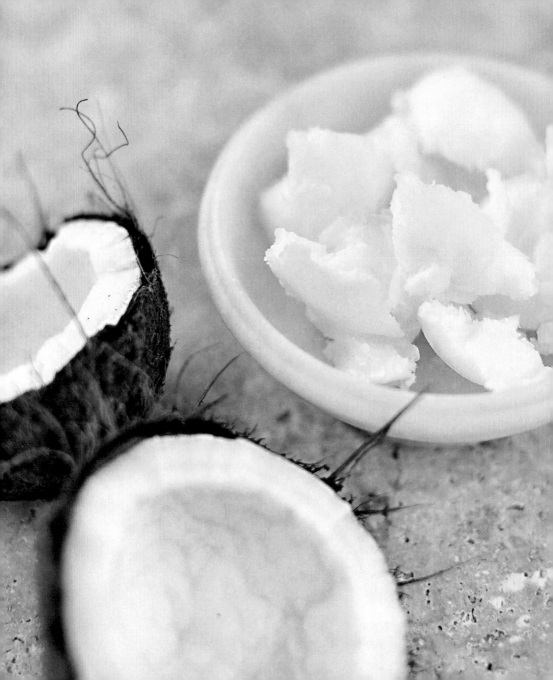

IT'S ALL ABOUT THE GLOW

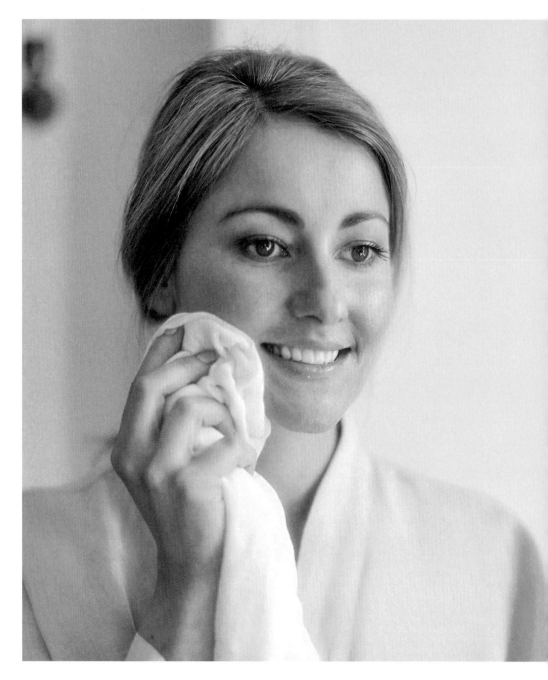

SHOW YOUR SKIN SOME LOVE

Who else wants their skin to be in the best condition it can be? Silly question, we all want that. As a beauty therapist I have heard all the concerns people have about their skin and how they want it to look plump, glowing, hydrated, youthful and, of course, how they want to get rid of those wrinkles and fine lines. Well, I have some great news for you: this book will help bring you one step closer to getting on the right track to a healthy new you, not only from the outside but from the inside too, with tips and tricks throughout the book.

DOUBLE CLEANSE DAILY

I feel it's best we start with something that we should really be doing twice a day (morning and night) and that is cleansing. This is important for everyone but especially if you live in a town or city, because when you cleanse you are washing away the pollution that ages skin. It also unclogs pores and prevents breakouts. The biggest culprits are soot and exhaust fumes, which are really good at getting into skin, where they trigger genes responsible for wrinkles and age spots (those brown clover-like clusters that appear on the cheeks, forehead, and bridge of the nose).

It's a bit like brushing your teeth – cleanse twice a day to help remove the impurities that build up on your face so less of them penetrate your skin.

Coconut oil is a very gentle way to cleanse because it dissolves stubborn make-up and binds to the pollution on your face so you can wash it away. Try the 'double-cleansing' method before bed, which is: apply one layer of coconut oil to remove make-up along with the dirt and pollution that are stuck to it. Rinse, then apply a second layer, working a warm, wet flannel in a circular motion over your face to deep-cleanse pores, buff away dead skin, and make skin look immediately brighter.

MOISTURIZE WITH OILS

For this section, you need to think of your skin as a wall. Your cells are the bricks and in between them are fats (similar to mortar) that keep water in the skin so it stays plump and moist. As we age, these fats break down; water starts to escape, skin becomes drier and wrinkles look deeper. So it's important to get into the habit of using plant oils such as coconut oil on your skin.

Most creams contain a little oil but not enough to make a big difference in water loss. Coconut oil, however, is fat-loving (or lipophilic to be exact) – meaning it passes through the surface of the skin more effectively, preventing water loss and keeping skin well hydrated.

DO FACIAL MASSAGE

Walking out of a treatment room after a facial not only makes us feel relaxed and pampered but you've probably also noticed that healthy pink glow on your cheeks, along with the definition of cheek bones slightly showing and any puffiness around your eyes and cheeks reduced. This is all down to facial massage. This increases blood flow, which can cause the skin to look brighter. It also encourages toxins to move to the lymph nodes, which helps with dark circles under the eyes and breaks up blocked sinuses that cause puffiness and headaches. Facial massage also has a firming and sculpting effect on your muscles – the scaffolding that supports your skin – that really makes your face look younger. Our pictures show how to do this – don't be put off, it's really simple and works incredibly well!

Do this as often as possible, with or without oil. My top tip is while watching the TV – you'll forget you're even doing it!

>>>

JUST USE COCONUT OIL!

1 STEP ONE: Warm the coconut oil in your hands and apply to your face.

2 STEP TWO: Your facial muscles are arranged diagonally in line with your cheekbones, so apply long strokes upwards to give them a workout and tighten up the skin.

3 STEP THREE: Lightly tap along the orbital bone (part of the eye socket) underneath your eye to get rid of puffiness. This will stimulate the lymphatic system, which lies just underneath the skin's surface and gets rid of excess fluid. Work from the inner corner of your eyes towards your ears, where the lymph nodes are located to flush it all out.

4 STEP FOUR: Pinch along your brows to release tension that leads to furrows and to stop the upper eyelids sagging.

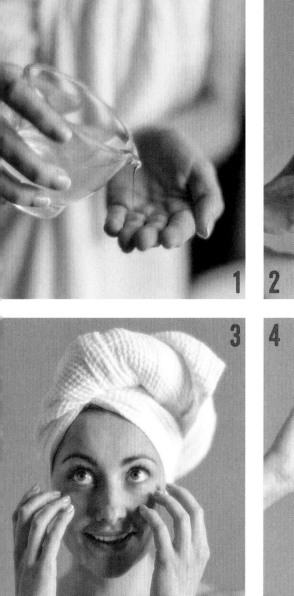
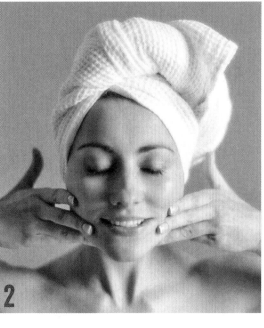
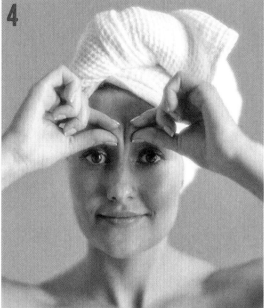

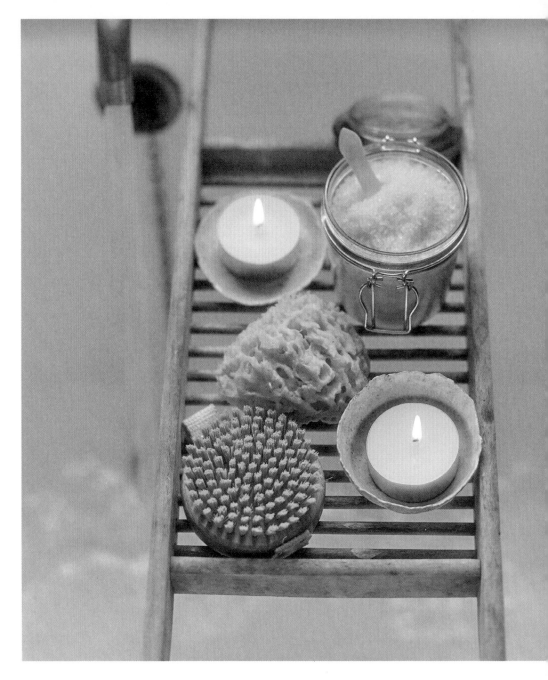

In an ideal world, stress would be banned! After all, what good does it bring anyone? None at all but sadly stress is a reality of everyday life. You can't avoid work, bills, or your daily commute so the best thing you can do is learn to manage it if you want to avoid throwing your body out of balance.

When we're anxious, our adrenal glands release adrenaline and cortisol. These two stress hormones increase sugar levels in the blood, causing insulin to be produced; this, in turn, triggers inflammation in the body linked to acne and eczema. Stress can also disrupt the balance between the good and bad bacteria in your gut, which shows up on your skin in the form of spots and rashes. It's also known that cortisol blocks the formation of collagen, the main protein that makes skin plump and bouncy.

Where possible try taking 20 minutes out of your busy day for relaxing 'me time', as this can work wonders emotionally and physically. Studies have shown that massaging your face and body lowers levels of these stress hormones and releases feel-good endorphins in your body. Meanwhile, slipping into a lukewarm bath is proven to be deeply relaxing and increases lymph flow, causing blood to rush to the skin's surface, drawing inflammation away from tensed up muscles.

'A RELAXING BATH IS THE PERFECT WAY TO UNWIND AFTER A BUSY DAY. TRY TO TAKE SOME TIME OUT OF EACH DAY TO CONCENTRATE ON ME TIME.'

GET YOUR ZZZS

Beauty sleep – there's a reason they call it this. Little did you know, when you're sleeping and unaware of what's going on, your skin is working hard to renew cells eight times faster than when awake and apparently the prime time for this is between 11pm and 3am!

New research has found that it's not just good enough to be in bed in time for a good eight hours' kip. The quality of your sleep makes a big difference to how well your skin renews itself overnight. Broken sleep – where you doze, toss, and turn – can interrupt these important processes. More worrying yet, a bad night's sleep can result in raised levels of the stress hormone cortisol, which can trigger skin issues to flare up.

Create a relaxing environment in your bedroom by switching off any electrical devices an hour before you go to sleep as the light from your smart phone or tablet simulates sunlight. If you struggle to nod off because your mind is busy rattling off tomorrow's to-do list, keep a notepad by your bed to jot down anything you are worrying you'll forget, so you don't have to think about it until the morning. Another great thing to try is a combination of aromatherapy, deep breathing, and visualisation: sprinkle a few drops of lavender essential oil on your pillowcase; close your eyes and take deep breaths in through your nose and out through your mouth. Then think of your favourite holiday spot or a place you relax – really visualize it and just enjoy the sensation of being there.

EXERCISE

Believe it or not, with every heart-pumping workout, your skin becomes more radiant. Exercise gets blood pumping around the body and makes your 2 million-plus sweat glands work harder. When you sweat, your pores become dilated, helping to flush out dead skin cells and bacteria and other skin-clogging nasties, so your complexion immediately looks brighter. It also helps boost your feel-good endorphins, so it's a win-win really... now to actually do the workout!

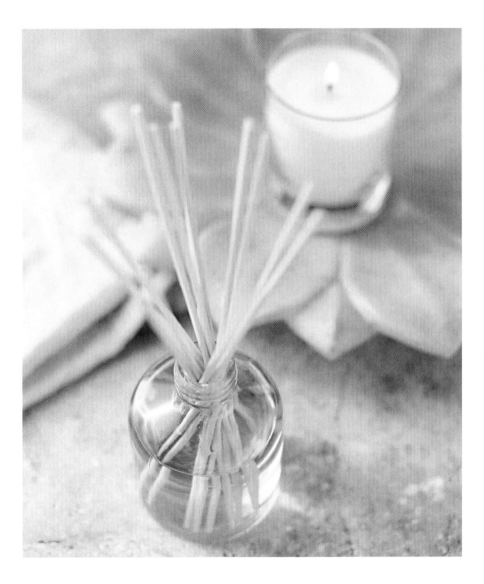

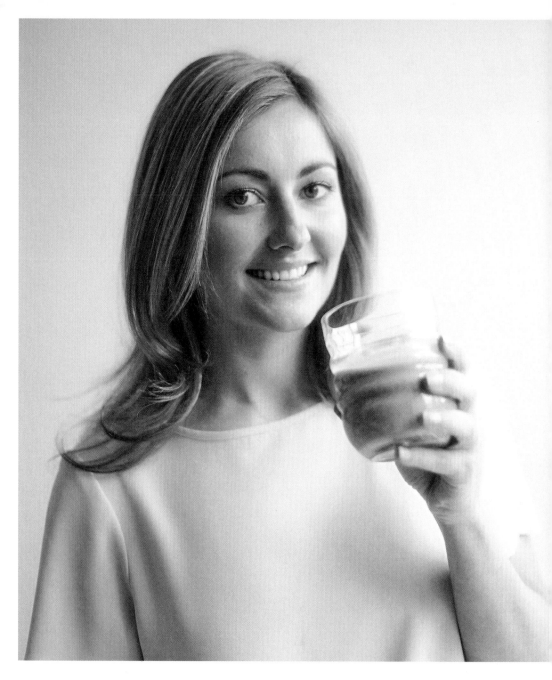

THE 'S' WORD

Sugar. You've no doubt read recent articles in the media confirming that sugar is the enemy in the fight against weight gain and good fats are actually our friend. Sugar is just as bad for your skin as it is for your waistline. When you ingest sugar, two things happen: firstly your body breaks it down into glucose, raising your insulin levels. The result is a burst of inflammation throughout the body, sometimes causing acne and eczema, amongst other things.

Secondly, a natural process known as glycation is set in motion – this is when the sugar in your bloodstream attaches itself to collagen and elastin, the proteins that keep skin firm and elastic. Once damaged, springy collagen and elastin become dry and brittle and can lead to wrinkles and sagging. Cut back on the sweet stuff and increase the number of antioxidant-rich fruits, nuts, good fats, and vegetables in your diet, as they help prevent sugar from attaching to your collagen and elastin. For more inspiration, check out my antioxidant-rich juices on page 24.

'DRINKING HOMEMADE JUICES IS A GREAT WAY TO MAKE SURE THAT YOU'RE GETTING PLENTY OF VITAMIN-RICH FRUIT AND VEGETABLES INTO YOUR DIET.'

FEED YOUR FACE

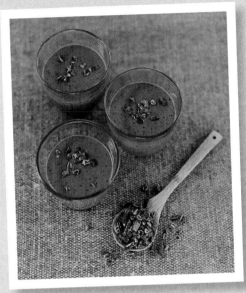

AVOCADO AND SPINACH SMOOTHIE
(Serves 1)

> Handful of spinach
> ½ avocado
> Seeds from 2 lightly crushed
  cardamom pods
> 250ml (8 fl. oz./1 cup) coconut water
> 10g (⅓ oz./1 tbsp) oats
> 2 Medjool dates, stones removed

Place all the ingredients in a blender
and blend together. Serve straight away,
with ice if preferred.

APPLE, BEETROOT AND ORANGE JUICE
(Serves 1)

> 1 apple
> 1 slice or ½ lemon (to taste)
> Small handful of parsley
> 1 small beetroot (beet), peeled
> 2 celery sticks
> ½ orange, peeled

Rinse all the ingredients well. Add each
ingredient to your juicer and enjoy.

CHOCOLATE SMOOTHIE FIX
(Serves 1)

> 50g (2 oz./⅔ cup) blueberries
> 1 ripe banana
> 250ml (8 fl. oz./1 cup) almond milk
> 1 tbsp Lucy Bee cacao powder
> 1 tsp peanut butter
> 1 tsp cacao nibs (optional)

Place all the ingredients except the cacao
nibs in a blender and blend together.
To serve, top with cacao nibs, if using.

TIP >>>
You could make a juice the night before
and keep in the refrigerator.

CARROT, CUCUMBER AND GINGER JUICE

(Serves 1)

> 2 carrots
> Handful of spinach
> 2cm (1 in.) piece of fresh ginger
> ½ cucumber
> 1 apple

Rinse all the ingredients well. Add each ingredient to your juicer, then serve as it is, or with ice.

LUCY BEE HOT CHOCOLATE

(Serves 1)

> 250ml (8 fl. oz./1 cup) almond milk or regular milk
> 1 tbsp Lucy Bee cacao powder
> ½ tsp Lucy Bee cinnamon powder (optional)

Put the ingredients into a saucepan and warm gently over a medium heat for 2–3 minutes, stirring occasionally, until heated through. For a nice, frothy result, whisk it or whiz it in a blender.

ALMOND MILK CHAI TEA WITH CARDAMOM

(Serves 4)

> 375ml (12 fl. oz/1½ cups) water
> 1 cinnamon stick
> Seeds from 5 lightly crushed cardamom pods
> 3 cloves
> 5cm (2 in.) piece of fresh ginger, peeled and quartered
> ¼ vanilla pod (bean), split lengthways and seeds scraped out
> 1 tbsp honey
> 2 black tea bags
> 375ml (12 fl. oz./1½ cups) almond milk
> Lucy Bee cinnamon powder, to serve

Bring the water and spices (including the scraped out piece of vanilla pod) to the boil in a small saucepan, then simmer for 12–15 minutes.

Stir in the honey and drop the tea bags in. Take off the heat, let it sit for 4 minutes, then strain through a fine strainer into your serving pot. Heat the almond milk in the same pan over a medium heat then pour into the tea and stir well. Sprinkle over a dusting of cinnamon and serve.

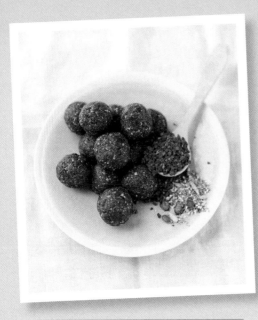

into a golf ball-sized ball, and place on a lined baking tray, then repeat with the remaining mixture. Place in the freezer for at least an hour, before storing in the freezer. I like to eat mine straight from the freezer.

LUCY BEE-TROOT HUMMUS WITH GARLIC
(Serves 6 as a dip)

> 300g (10½ oz.) raw beetroot (beet), chopped into small pieces
> 1 or 2 garlic cloves, chopped
> 1 tsp Lucy Bee coconut oil, melted
> 1 x 400g (15 oz.) can chickpeas (garbanzo beans), drained
> 60g (2 oz./¼ cup) tahini
> Juice of 1½ lemons
> 70ml (2½ fl. oz./⅓ cup) extra virgin olive oil
> A pinch of Lucy Bee Himalayan salt and ground black pepper

RASPBERRY FRUIT BITES WITH FLAXSEEDS
(Makes 12)

> 75g (2½ oz./¾ cup) mixed dried fruit and berries (I use a mixture containing cranberries, goji berries, and raisins)
> 40g (1½ oz./4 tbsp) Lucy Bee coconut oil, melted
> 75g (2½ oz./½ cup) dates
> 75g (2½ oz./½ cup) dried apricots
> 100g (3½ oz./¾ cup) flaxseeds
> 10g (⅓ oz./2 tbsp) freeze-dried raspberry powder
> 1 tsp Lucy Bee maca powder

Place all the ingredients in a food processor and blend until you have a doughy mixture. Take a teaspoon of the mixture, roll it

Preheat the oven to 170°C/325°F/gas mark 3. Mix the beetroot (beet) and garlic with the melted coconut oil in a roasting tray and roast in the oven for 30 minutes. Once cooked and softened, transfer to a food processor with the chickpeas (garbanzo beans), tahini, lemon juice, and oil and blitz to a fine paste – you may need to add a little more lemon juice or oil to get your desired consistency. Stir in salt and pepper to taste and serve with chopped carrots, celery, and cucumber, or pitta bread. It will keep for up to 5 days in the refrigerator.

WINTER SALAD

(Serves 1)

> 1 small sweet potato, peeled and diced
> 1 tbsp Lucy Bee coconut oil, melted
> Sprinkling of nigella seeds
> 1 salmon fillet
> 4 asparagus spears, each broken into 3
> 10g (⅓ oz./1 tbsp) pumpkin seeds
> Handful of rocket (arugula) leaves
> 30g (1 oz./¼ cup) soft goat cheese, chopped into small cubes
> 80g (3 oz.) cherry tomatoes, halved
> 5g (¼ oz./⅛ cup) chives, finely sliced

For the dressing
> 1 tbsp extra virgin olive oil
> 1 tbsp apple cider vinegar
> 1½ tbsp coconut aminos (or tamari if unavailable)
> 1 tbsp honey
> 2cm (1 in.) piece of fresh ginger

Preheat the oven to 180°C/350°F/gas mark 4. Put the sweet potato and melted coconut oil in a bowl and mix in the nigella seeds. Spread out on a roasting tray and roast in the oven for 10 minutes, then remove from the oven, add the salmon fillet and asparagus to the tray and place back in the oven for a further 15 minutes, by which time the sweet potatoes should be soft, and the salmon and asparagus both cooked. Set aside.

While the salmon and veg are cooking, make the dressing by blitzing all the ingredients together. Toast the pumpkin seeds in a dry frying pan (skillet) over a medium-high heat until they pop, then tip onto a small plate.

Place the rocket (arugula) leaves on a serving plate and top with the sweet potato, asparagus, goat cheese, and tomatoes, placing the salmon alongside. Scatter the pumpkin seeds and pour the dressing over the salad. Sprinkle the chives over everything to serve.

SUMMER SALAD

(Serves 1)

> 1 small beetroot (beet), cooked and cubed
> 1 medium carrot, peeled and grated
> 1 small Romaine lettuce, thinly sliced
> 6cm (2¼ in.) piece of cucumber, deseeded and cut into small chunks
> Handful of mint leaves, finely sliced
> 30g (1 oz./¼ cup) feta, crumbled or diced
> 1 hard-boiled egg, quartered
> 4 anchovy fillets (canned), chopped

For the dressing
> 1 tbsp white wine vinegar
> 1 tbsp extra virgin olive oil
> 30g (1 oz./¼ cup) fresh or frozen raspberries, defrosted if frozen
> ½ tbsp honey

In a bowl, mix together the beetroot (beet), carrot, lettuce, cucumber, mint, and feta. Tip the mixture into a serving dish, top with the hard-boiled egg and place an anchovy fillet over each egg quarter. Put all the dressing ingredients in a food processor or blender and blitz, then pour over the salad to serve.

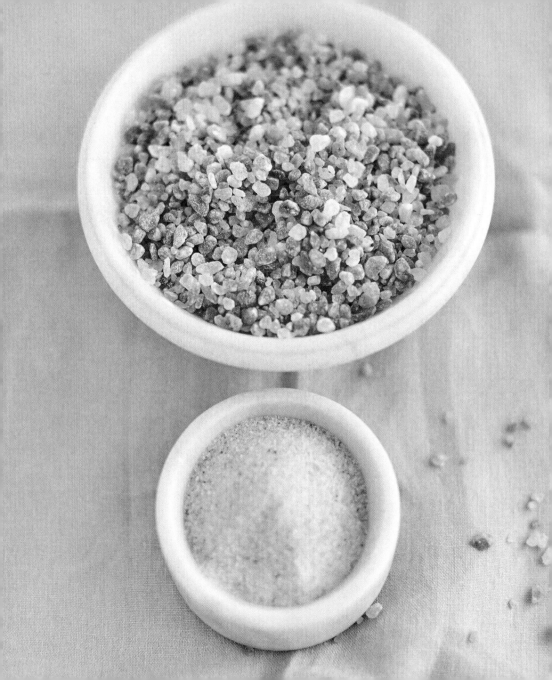

BEAUTY INGREDIENTS

SOME OF MY FAVOURITE THINGS

Nature provides us with an abundance of fruits, seeds, plants, and minerals that have incredible benefits for the skin. I'm a big fan of using those we keep stocked in the kitchen cupboard alongside hero ingredients from the plant world, many of which are widely recognized for their genuine effectiveness. The following crop up time and again in both my beauty and food recipes.

SUPERFOODS FOR GORGEOUS SKIN AND HAIR

Often the most effective beauty ingredients are found in the simplest of places: the nectar collected by bees and a plant's oils, butters, and roots.

COCONUT OIL

There are few beauty cure-alls but in my experience coconut oil comes pretty close. I use my extra virgin raw coconut oil as an alternative to traditional cooking oils, but you can put that jar to good use in your beauty routine, too.

Extracted from the meat of mature coconuts, coconut oil is primarily composed of fatty acids, which hydrate the skin by trapping water in the layers where it needs it most and which also reduce inflammation. When it comes to softening rough, leathery skin anywhere on the body, there's no competition. Chronic skin conditions such as eczema benefit, too. Coconut oil is predominantly made up of lauric acid (approximately 48%), known for its antifungal and antibacterial properties, so along with lessening inflammation, it prevents infection from scratching at the skin. To aid in your anti-ageing quest, coconut oil has been shown to be an effective antioxidant, using ferulic acid to shield against wrinkle-causing pollutants and other environment aggressors.

Coconut oil can feed your hair as well. When warmed from a solid to a liquid, it penetrates strands better than any other oil, smoothing away brittleness and helping to relieve the scaly skin linked to dandruff. Better yet, you'll smell like a tropical holiday even when skies are grey!

MELTING COCONUT OIL >>>

A lot of the recipes in this book use coconut oil in its liquid state. The easiest way to melt solid coconut oil is to place a glass heatproof bowl inside a saucepan filled with enough water to touch the base of the bowl. Scoop the solid coconut oil into the bowl and warm over a medium heat until it turns to a liquid.

SHEA BUTTER

Shea butter is an incredible moisturizer used for centuries by women in sub-Saharan Africa to nourish and protect their skin and hair. It is a natural fat extracted from the nut of the shea tree and has one of the richest concentrations of fatty acids – the same natural moisturizers that your skin's sebaceous glands produce. Shea butter is also bursting with anti-inflammatory vitamin E and vitamin A, known to aid in treating blemishes, wrinkles, and eczema.

Like coconut oil, shea butter is solid at room temperature but melts on contact with the skin to produce a lightweight oil that dry or sensitive skin immediately drinks up.

HONEY

Honey is so much more than just a natural sweetener or breakfast condiment for spreading on toast. Raw honey, which hasn't been heat-treated or pasteurized, contains a host of active nutrients and enzymes that nourish and heal the skin.

First and foremost, honey is a natural humectant, meaning it draws moisture from the air into the skin and hydrates deep down. Honey is also a useful ingredient in conditioner as it locks moisture in the hair and gives dull strands added shine. Honey's other big draws are its antibacterial properties, which thwart acne-causing bacteria and its anti-inflammatory compounds that calm irritation and increase healing in fresh scar tissue.

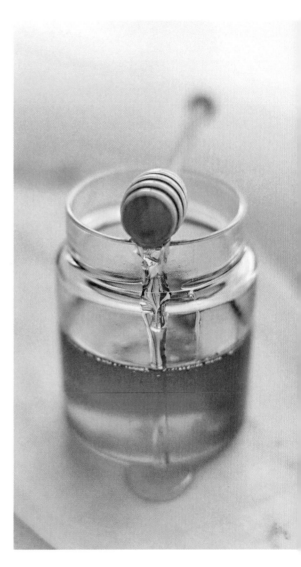

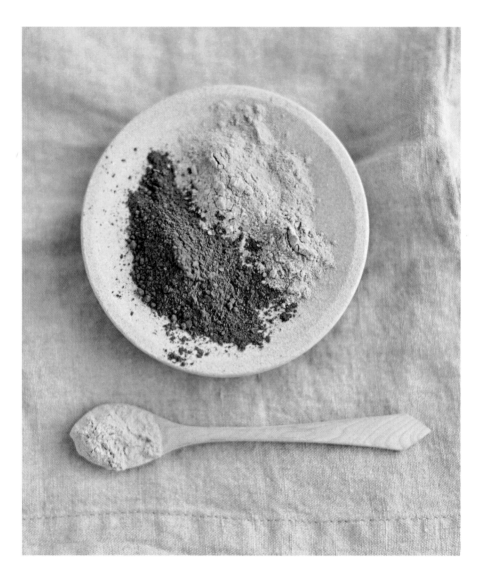

CACAO

Raw cacao (pronounced 'ca-cow') is one of the purest forms of chocolate. It contains more than 300 nutritional compounds, making it one of the best sources of antioxidants on the planet. Incredibly, raw cacao contains 20 times the number of antioxidants found in blueberries and nearly four times more than standard dark chocolate.

Lucy Bee cacao is made from a rare breed of Criollo and Forastero beans grown in the mineral-rich soil of the Dominican Republic. The pods grow directly from the tree trunks and turn an orange or yellow colour as they ripen before being hand-picked and placed in cedar boxes to ferment. After two days the cocoa beans are roasted below 45°C/ 113°F to retain their rawness and maximum nutritional value, then the fat (or butter) is stripped away.

Fair Trade and supporting our producer countries and farmers is something I'm extremely passionate about. Through our Fair Trade contributions, our producers in the Dominican Republic plan to set up a Copay Fund to help pay for essential medical visits and treatment for the single mums who harvest our cacao, as well as enabling their children to learn English and so help their future work prospects.

MACA

Growing at altitudes of over 4,200m (14,000 feet) in the Peruvian Andes, maca (also known as Peruvian ginseng) may be relatively new to us but it's been used as a herbal remedy for thousands of years. Maca is an adaptogen, a herb used to help the body deal with stressful events. There are also numerous claims of it being a physical and mental health source of energy, which supports performance, hormone balance, and vitality. According to legend, Inca warriors would take maca before battles to improve their fighting spirit. It's not surprising then, that these days maca is used in smoothies for added energy.

But maca is also becoming increasingly known as a beauty all-rounder. It is rich in brightening vitamin C and contains high levels of copper, known to improve skin elasticity, firmness, and thickness.

Lucy Bee's maca is sown by hand and fertilized naturally, without the use of pesticides and chemicals and is watered by natural rainfall. When the maca root is ready for harvesting, it is hand-picked and dried in the sun for 20–30 days. Then, using the traditional Peruvian method of gelatinisation, the starch is removed before the root is milled into a fine powder. The result? 100% pure maca and the very best we've ever tried.

BEAUTY SALTS

Whether pouring into a bath or using to make a homemade body scrub, Himalayan, Dead Sea, and Epsom salts will get you through those busy, stressful days and replenish your skin's lost minerals.

DEAD SEA SALTS

For centuries, the Dead Sea has been renowned for its healing properties. Since Roman times, people have flocked to bathe in its waters to relieve muscular tension and joint pain and to treat skin conditions such as eczema.

Containing up to eight times more minerals than regular sea water, the Dead Sea is the saltiest in the world, which is why you can float in it. And it's these salts that are key to our health and wellbeing. Lucy Bee's Dead Sea salts contain 21 minerals, including magnesium, potassium, and calcium chloride, to balance skin moisture and ease muscle stiffness. They are gathered from the sea and hand-picked before being washed and dried. The granules are then sieved and separated according to their various sizes for use as bath salts and exfoliating scrubs.

HIMALAYAN SALT

With its delicate shade of baby pink, this crystal salt is considered so precious a commodity it is known as the 'salt of life' and even the 'King's salt' because at one time it was reserved only for royalty. The salt itself began life over 250 million years ago as a crystallized sea salt bed within the Himalayan mountains. Covered in lava, it is protected against modern-day pollution, making Himalayan salt the purest in the world. Today, Lucy Bee's Himalayan salt continues to be mined from these ancient crystal salt deposits. Its 84 natural trace minerals, including calcium, iron, and magnesium, are packed in a colloidal form (which basically means they're teeny tiny), so the goodness is easily absorbed by your body's cells.

EPSOM SALTS

While they may seem like a new-fangled, fashionable must-have for reducing water retention and tummy bloating, Epsom salts are in fact an age-old home remedy. First discovered in the 17th century by a farmer in Epsom, Surrey (hence the name), the salt was originally formed in saline springs and fast became a natural remedy for aches and pains.

Modern Epsom salts like ours are made from a rock substance called dolomite, found in the mountainous regions of the Southern Alps. Essentially a mix of magnesium, sulphates, and regular old oxygen, the minerals and elements in these salts can be absorbed by the skin's pores when bathing or exfoliating. Magnesium is a mineral many people are deficient in, even though it's the second most abundant element in our cells. As the magnesium is absorbed into the skin, activating the body's healing mechanisms, a form of reverse osmosis occurs and any toxins and excess fluids are drawn out of the skin.

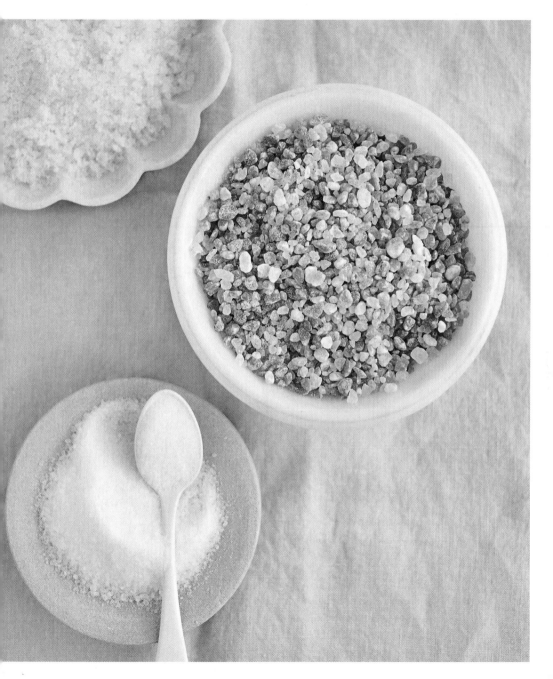

Essential oils are a natural fragrant extracted from plants. I love adding them to my beauty recipes as they are very clever in the way they work. Not only do they all have distinctive smells, they are also known for their incredible properties. To name a few of their benefits: they can be used to revitalize; stimulate; de-stress; soothe; and help with depression, sleepless nights, and even illness.

LAVENDER (Lavendula angustifolia)

The sweet-scented, purple-flowered bush has a long history as a medicinal herb. At one time, people used lavender oil to ward off the plague and its antiseptic and anti-inflammatory properties meant that in the First World War, lavender was used on soldiers' wounds. Even now, lavender oil can be used to soothe acne and other skin complaints. But it is lavender's profound effect on stress levels that makes it such a popular essential oil. Scientists have proved that a whiff of lavender triggers alpha waves in the brain, lowering stress hormones, slowing down heart rate, and calming the nervous system.

ROSE (Rosa centifolia)

For aromatherapy, the essential oil extract from a rose's velvety petals is believed to have calming, antidepressant benefits. It's known to help lift your spirits on days when you're thinking the glass is half empty and evokes feelings of nostalgia that bring to mind happy memories. Applied topically, it's ideal for dry and ageing skin. Rose oil is rich in hydrating essential fatty acids to restore softness to your skin. It's particularly good for people with thread veins and sensitivity as it helps to strengthen and calm the skin and take away redness.

LEMON (Citrus limonum)

Extracted from the rind, lemon oil has a sharp, invigorating scent that scientists have found improves mental accuracy and concentration – perfect if you've hit that 3pm slump in energy levels. Its stimulating power extends to the body, too. Lemon oil can help to kick-start the lymphatic system, responsible for flushing out toxins and excess fluid, which is why you'll often find it in body-toning oils and creams. Lemon oil is also bursting with antibacterial and antifungal properties, making it an ideal natural alternative for treating pimples and reducing excessive sebum on the skin.

PEPPERMINT (Mentha x piperita)

The menthol in peppermint creates a cooling effect on the skin, which makes it useful for easing muscular pains and headaches when rubbed onto the forehead and temples. Added to beauty products, peppermint oil instantly freshens and revives the skin. It is known to have astringent properties, helping to normalize the amount of oil on the skin's surface. Preparations containing peppermint oil are also useful for treating a dry scalp and dandruff as it helps to heal the skin and prevents itching, too.

TEA TREE *(Melaleuca alternifolia)*

The name 'tea tree' was coined by British explorer James Cook in the 1770s, when he witnessed aboriginal communities brewing tea using the leaves from the tree and applying it as an antiseptic for treating skin conditions. Modern science has revealed that 40% of tea tree oil is made up of the antibacterial compound called terpinen-4-ol. This explains why it is useful for treating moderate acne and also has antifungal benefits for treating dandruff.

ROSEMARY *(Rosmarinus officinalis)*

Rosemary, with its greyish green, needle-shaped leaves, is an aromatic herb with a clean, woody aroma. When the oil is inhaled, it is known to clear the respiratory tract. Worked into aching joints and tensed up muscles, its anti-inflammatory properties kick in and offer relief from pain. But it is in hair care that rosemary oil is most widely used. Massaging the scalp with rosemary oil dilates the blood vessels and stimulates the follicles. This encourages new hair growth and helps existing strands to grow longer and stronger.

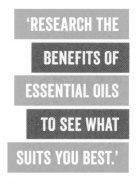

'RESEARCH THE BENEFITS OF ESSENTIAL OILS TO SEE WHAT SUITS YOU BEST.'

PATCH TESTING >>>

When trying a product for the first time, it is a good idea to do a patch test. Apply sparingly to a small area of skin behind your ear and wait 24 hours to make sure there are no adverse reactions.

GLASS BOWL AND SAUCEPAN

Most of my recipes involve liquefying coconut oil. A simple way to do this is to place a glass heatproof bowl inside a saucepan (see page 30).

MEDIUM-SIZED MIXING BOWL

You'll need this when mixing up coconut oil or stirring together different ingredients.

SIEVE AND MUSLIN CLOTH

These can be used to filter your beauty products when a smooth texture is required.

HAND-HELD MIXER

Use to beat the oils until they are fluffy, like whipped cream.

GLASS JARS AND CONTAINERS IN VARIOUS SIZES

These are perfect for storing all your lovely homemade beauty products.

DRY BRUSH

Before applying any of my body products, use a dry brush to stimulate blood flow. Brush lightly in an upward motion, starting from the soles of your feet, up your legs, back and arms, always working in the direction of your heart.

TRY THIS! >>>

Dry brushing is great for circulation and can help with the appearance of cellulite too. Brush for 1 minute in strokes towards the heart. Do this morning and night before getting in the shower and then apply nourishing coconut oil.

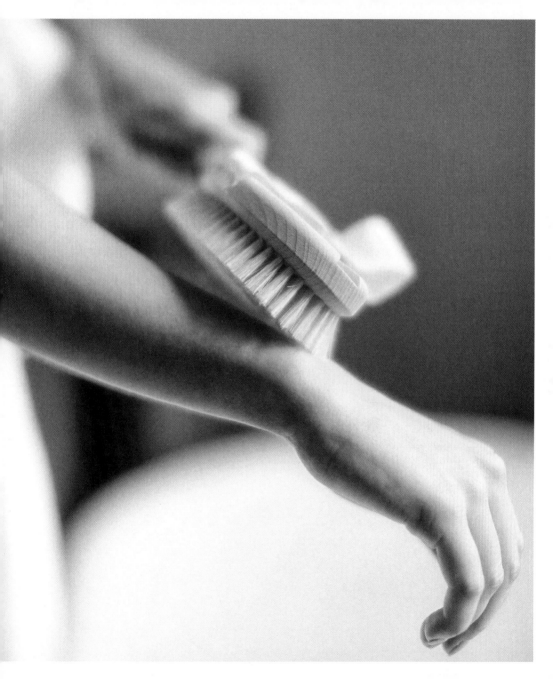

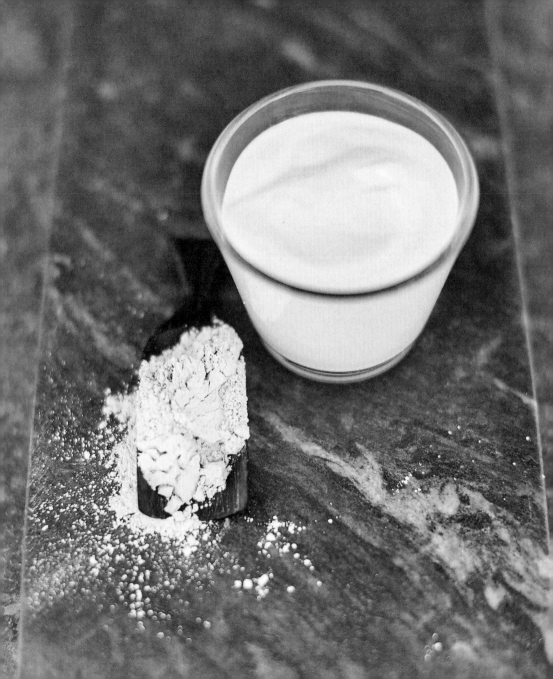

FOR THE FACE

HONEY AND COCONUT OIL CLEANSER

(Makes 1 x 80ml or 3 fl. oz. jar)

The beauty of this cleanser is that it's gentle but still packs a punch by only containing three of the best antibacterial ingredients from the natural world: coconut oil, honey, and lavender.

> 50g (2 oz./5 tbsp) Lucy Bee coconut oil, melted
> 2 tbsp honey
> 5 drops lavender essential oil

Pour the coconut oil into a small mixing bowl. Stir in the honey and lavender oil and combine thoroughly. Leave to cool before using or transferring to a jar. Use a tablespoon-sized dollop on dry skin morning and night.

TRY THIS! >>>

Apply one layer of neat coconut oil to remove your make-up (see page 55). After wiping it away with a damp cotton pad, apply this cleanser. This time, take a few minutes to rub the cleanser in circular motions all over your face and neck, giving yourself a gentle massage as you go. Use a warm, wet flannel to lift away the residue.

HIMALAYAN SALT EXFOLIATOR

(Makes enough for 1 use)

Exfoliating your face unclogs pores, restores lustre to even the dullest complexion, and speeds up skin renewal by allowing new healthy cells to replace dead ones on the skin's surface.

> ½ tsp Lucy Bee Himalayan salt
> 1 tbsp Honey and Coconut Oil Cleanser (see left)

Add the Himalayan salt to the Honey and Coconut Oil Cleanser and use once a week, working the mixture into your skin using a circular motion, to remove dead skin cells, then rinse.

ALMOND MILK CLEANSER

(Makes about 250ml or 8½ fl. oz.)

> 25g (1 oz./¼ cup) ground almonds
> 1 tbsp honey
> 250ml (8 fl. oz./1 cup) bottled water

Add the ground almonds and honey to the bottled water and stir well until the honey has dissolved. Leave to rest for 2 hours. To filter, pour through a muslin-lined sieve into a covered container or bottle and store in a refrigerator. Apply generously to the face and neck using a cotton wool ball and leave for 20 minutes – time for the lotion to penetrate the skin and dry naturally. This will keep in the refrigerator for up to 4 days.

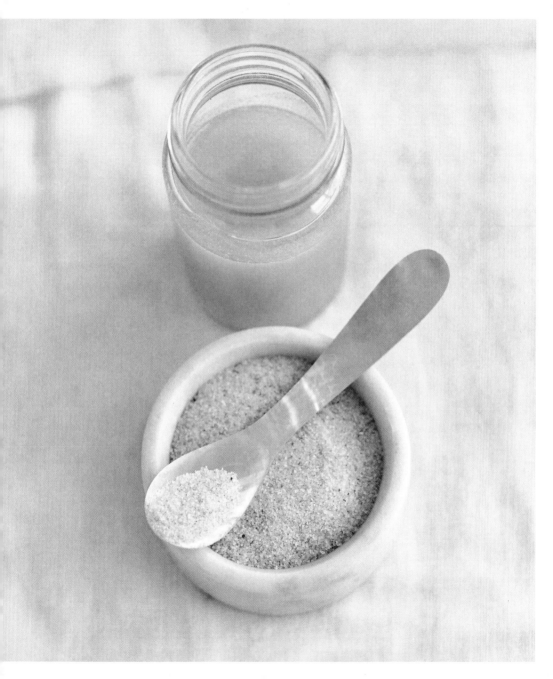

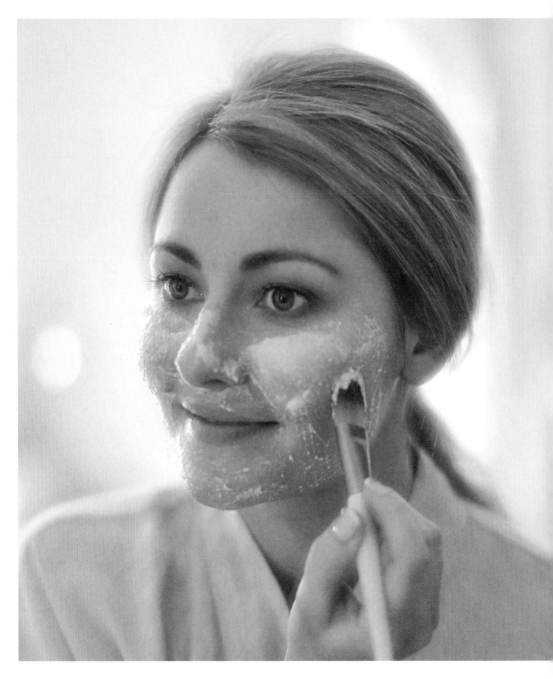

AVOCADO AND EVENING PRIMROSE FACE MASK

(Makes 1 mask)

> ½ very ripe small avocado
> 1 tsp Lucy Bee coconut oil, melted
> 1 tsp natural (plain) live yogurt
> 1 capsule evening primrose oil

Mash the avocado flesh using the back of a fork and add to a small mixing bowl. Add the melted coconut oil and yogurt. Snip or prick open the evening primrose oil capsule and squeeze the contents into the bowl, stirring well to mix. If the mixture seems very lumpy, you can press it through a sieve. Apply evenly to the cleaned face and neck, avoiding the eye area, and leave for 20 minutes. Rinse with water and cotton wool balls and pat dry.

HONEY AND CITRUS RADIANCE FACE MASK

(Makes 1 mask)

Coconut oil and honey are moisturizing powerhouses but throw in orange juice, with its burst of vitamin C, and you've got the recipe for an instant glow. Apply after a late night to erase all signs of tiredness.

> 1 tsp Lucy Bee coconut oil, melted
> ½ tsp honey
> ½ tsp freshly squeezed orange juice

Pour the melted coconut oil into a small mixing bowl and add the honey and orange juice. Stir to mix and leave to cool before applying or transferring to a glass bottle. When ready to use, spread the mask onto your face and neck, avoiding the eye area, and leave for 20 minutes, then rinse off with warm water and pat the skin dry with a towel.

MACA AND CACAO BRIGHTENING FACE MASK

(Makes 1 mask)

Maca and cacao are antioxidant-filled superfoods, while clay is one of the best pore cleansers. Use twice weekly to banish dull, tired-looking skin and refine the look of pores.

> 2 tsp Lucy Bee coconut oil, melted
> 1 tsp Lucy Bee maca powder
> 1 tsp Lucy Bee cacao powder
> 1 tsp bentonite clay powder

Pour the coconut oil into a small mixing bowl. Stir in all the other ingredients until they form a paste. After cleansing and exfoliating, pat your face dry and spread the mask onto your face and neck, avoiding the eye area. Allow the mask to sit on your skin for 15–20 minutes. Gently rinse with warm water.

PINEAPPLE EXFOLIATING MASK

(Makes 1 mask)

> 1 tbsp fresh mint leaves
> 1 ripe very small pineapple
> 2–3 tbsp oatmeal

To make a mint infusion, place the mint leaves in a mug, fill with boiling water and leave for 10 minutes. Strain, then leave the liquid to cool. Peel the pineapple and cut it in half lengthways. Remove the pithy central section, using a knife or spoon, and purée it in a food processor or blender (save the flesh for eating). Stir 2 tbsp of the cooled mint infusion into the purée, mixing well, and then enough oatmeal to make a smooth paste. Apply to the face and neck, avoiding the area around the eyes, and leave for about 15 minutes. Remove with water, using cotton wool balls. Dab on some of the remaining mint infusion and leave to dry naturally.

YOGURT AND EVENING PRIMROSE MASK

(Makes 1 mask)

> 1 capsule evening primrose oil
> 1 capsule vitamin E oil
> 1 tbsp natural (plain) live yogurt
> 1 tsp honey
> About ½ tsp bentonite clay powder

Snip or prick open the evening primrose oil and vitamin E oil capsules and squeeze the contents into a small mixing bowl. Add the remaining ingredients and stir well. If the consistency is too runny, add a little more clay powder and stir again. Apply evenly to the cleansed face and neck, avoiding the area around the eyes, and leave for 20 minutes. Rinse off using water and cotton wool balls and pat dry.

RASPBERRY RIPPLE MASK

(Makes 1 mask)

> 7–8 ripe raspberries
> 1 tbsp natural (plain) live yogurt
> 1 tbsp honey
> 2 tsp bentonite clay powder

Mash the raspberries using the back of a fork, or purée them in a small food processor or blender. Add the yogurt, honey, and clay powder to the purée to form a thick mixture. Apply to the cleansed face and neck, avoiding the area around the eyes, and leave for about 10 minutes. Rinse off using water and cotton wool balls and pat dry.

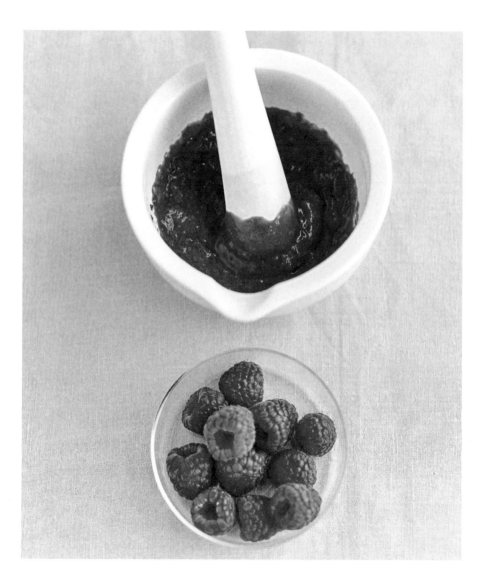

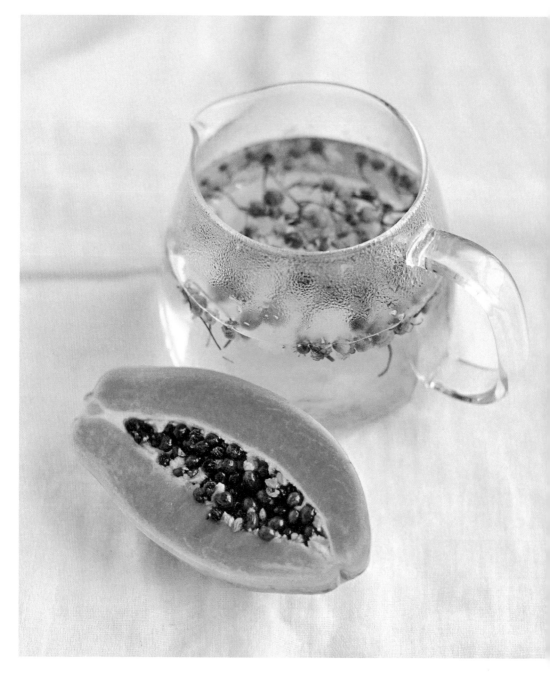

PAPAYA EXFOLIATING LOTION

(Makes 1 mask)

This is very good for blackheads. Use the smallest papaya that you can find!

> 1 small papaya
> About 250ml (8½ fl. oz/1 cup) chamomile infusion, cooled

Peel the papaya, remove the seeds, and purée the flesh in a food processor or blender. Mix the purée with an equal amount of chamomile infusion, stirring well. Using cotton wool balls, apply the lotion to the face and neck, avoiding any contact with the eyes. Leave for about 10 minutes then rinse off with water. Dab on a little of the remaining chamomile infusion, or some rosewater, and leave to dry naturally.

ANTI-BLEMISH FACE MASK

(Makes 1–2 masks)

Coconut oil and honey are both naturally antibacterial. The challenge is trying not to lick it off your face – let it do its work!

> 1 tbsp Lucy Bee coconut oil, melted
> 1 tsp honey

Pour the melted coconut oil into a small mixing bowl and stir in the honey. Leave to cool before using. Apply a thick layer to your face, avoiding contact with the eyes. Leave the mask on for 10 minutes, then rinse off with water.

SPIRULINA VITALIZING MASK

(Makes 1 mask)

> 1 tbsp spirulina powder
> 2 tbsp white or green clay powder
> 1 tbsp Lucy Bee coconut oil, melted
> 3 tbsp water

Mix the spirulina and clay powders together in a bowl. Add the melted coconut oil and stir to mix. Pour the water over and leave for 30 minutes without stirring, then mix well to form a smooth paste. Apply to the cleansed face and neck, avoiding the area around the eyes. Leave for 20 minutes then wash off with water, patting dry with cotton wool balls.

BROWN SUGAR LIP SCRUB

(Makes enough for 3–5 applications)

In winter, lips can easily get dry and chapped. To create a smooth surface for your lip balm – and to ensure it sinks in rather than clings to the dead skin – use this lip scrub as often as needed.

> 1 tsp Lucy Bee coconut oil
> 1 tsp brown sugar

Mash the coconut oil to a paste and mix in the brown sugar. Smear generously over the lips, massaging the gritty sugar granules into the skin in a circular motion. When finished, simply lick it off!

COCONUT OIL LIP BALM

(Makes enough for 10 applications)

Coconut oil is super hydrating but the fact it melts easily doesn't always make it the best thing to carry around with you. Adding beeswax keeps it solid – they are the perfect hydrating duo!

> 1 tbsp Lucy Bee coconut oil
> 1 tbsp beeswax

Place a glass heatproof bowl inside a saucepan filled with enough water to touch the base of the bowl. Scoop the solid coconut oil and beeswax into the bowl and warm over a medium heat until the mixture turns to a liquid. Remove from the heat and leave to cool before using or transferring to a glass container.

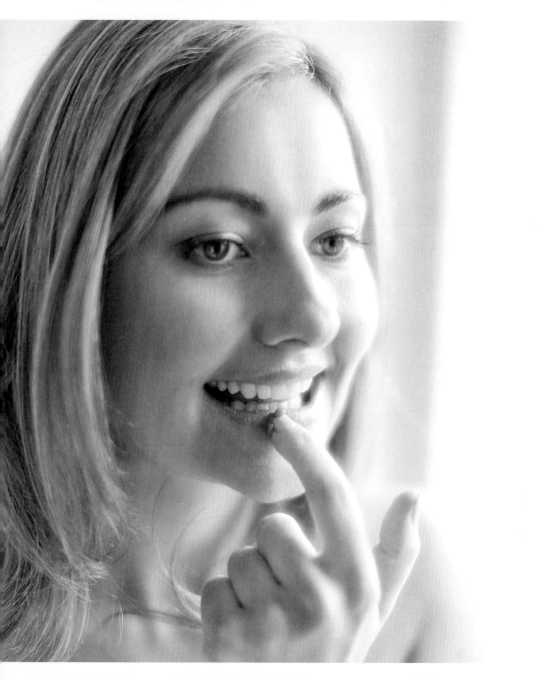

HOMEMADE ECZEMA CREAM

(Makes about 50g or 2 oz.)

Eczema is a condition where patches of skin become rough and inflamed, with blisters that cause itching and bleeding. We receive lots of messages from eczema sufferers, telling us how our raw coconut oil has helped soothe and heal their skin. If you suffer from eczema, I really hope this helps you too.

> 50g (2 oz./5 tbsp) Lucy Bee coconut oil, melted
> 1 tbsp honey
> 40 drops lavender essential oil
> 5–10 drops tea tree essential oil

Pour the melted coconut oil into a small mixing bowl and stir in the honey and essential oils. Leave to cool, then use a hand-held mixer to froth up the mixture until it has a texture similar to a lotion. Pour into a glass jar and store at room temperature, where it will solidify.

REJUVENATING NIGHT CREAM

(Makes 1 x 40g or 1½ oz. jar)

As we get older, the skin's protective outer layer, which keeps the layers beneath plump with water, weakens; skin becomes dehydrated and lines more prominent. Used on its own, coconut oil will drip-feed moisture into the skin. But for a more powerful rejuvenating hit, I've added rosehip oil and skin-softening vitamin E to the mixture. Yes, rosehip oil is pricey (in fact, it's the most expensive item in the book) but it's one of the most widely recognized sources of antioxidant vitamins and skin-nourishing essential fatty acids, important for keeping skin smooth, supple and protecting against ageing free radicals. A little goes a long way, too, so if you can, I'd recommend making the investment.

> 40g (1½ oz./4 tbsp) Lucy Bee coconut oil, melted
> 1 vitamin E capsule
> 2 tsp rosehip oil

Pour the melted coconut oil into a small mixing bowl. Break open the vitamin E capsule and empty the contents into the bowl, then stir in the rosehip oil. Leave to cool before applying or transferring to a glass jar or bottle. When ready to use, massage into your face before bed, taking it up around the eyes.

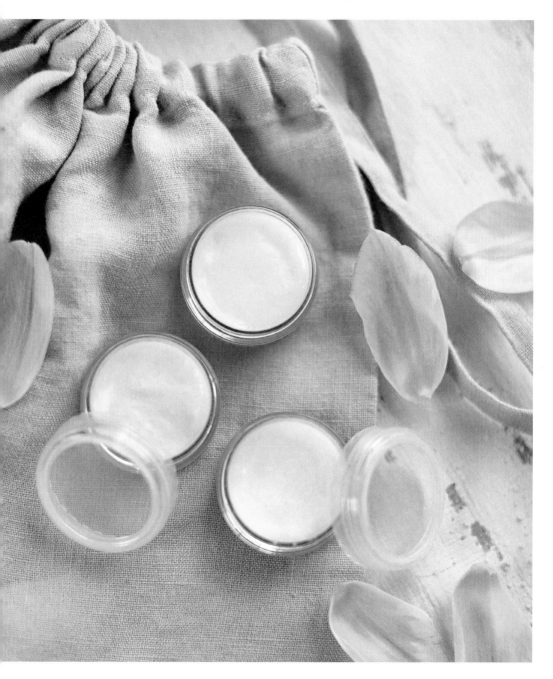

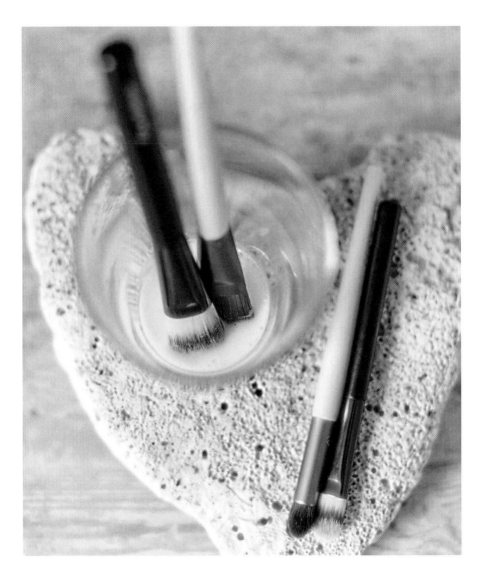

MAKE-UP BRUSH CLEANER

(Makes enough for 1 use)

Ideally you should clean your make-up brushes every two weeks to lift away the oil and dead skin cells embedded deep within the bristles. You don't want them to turn into breeding grounds for bacteria.

> 1 tbsp Lucy Bee coconut oil, melted
> 1 tbsp antibacterial soap

Pour the melted coconut oil into a small mixing bowl and stir in the antibacterial soap. Leave to cool then massage into the bristles of your brushes. Avoid the barrel – if it gets wet, this can cause the bristles to loosen and fall out. Rinse the brushes and place on their sides on a flat towel to dry (if you stand them up, the water will run down into the handle and cause rust).

MAKE-UP REMOVER

(Makes enough for 1 use)

Even the most resistant waterproof mascara doesn't stand a chance against coconut oil. It's brilliant for breaking down the waxes used in make-up products without stinging your eyes.

> ½ tsp Lucy Bee coconut oil

Simply warm the solid coconut oil between your palms until it starts to liquefy. Then massage over your skin. Use a damp cotton wool pad to remove the oil and any make-up. It doesn't get much easier than this!

JUST USE COCONUT OIL!

SIMPLE TIPS FOR A HEALTHIER YOU

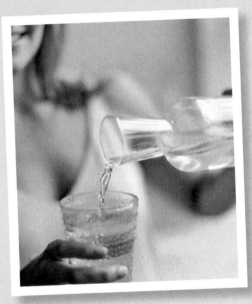

START EACH DAY WITH A GLASS OF WARM WATER WITH LEMON JUICE AND FRESH GINGER

This is great for detoxing your digestive system and removing accumulated waste products from your body, which is why I like to have this every morning after oil pulling (see page 83). You may be surprised to learn that although lemons are very acidic, when digested they become alkaline, helping to balance the body's pH levels.

PHONE SCREEN SAVER

This one may seem quite random but I find it really useful to write down my goals in my notepad on my phone, screenshot it, and then make it my background. For example, drinking 2 litres (1¾ quarts) of water per day or doing 100 squats a day (nice try, Lucy!). It might sound silly but it really works for me.

GET SOME FRESH AIR

Not only is this a great way to clear the mind and get a natural glow but it's also a great excuse to meet up with a friend and have a good catch up while you walk or run together!

NO CAFFEINE AFTER LUNCH

I have mentioned the importance of a good night's sleep for your skin, so avoiding caffeine after midday is a must.

AFTER A LONG DAY

Take a 20 minute soak in a Lucy Bee salt (Epsom, Himalayan or Dead Sea) bath with a dollop of Lucy Bee coconut oil; your skin and tired muscles will love you for the magnesium fix.

PREP AND PLAN YOUR MEALS

Being organized is a must with a busy life. Planning meals and preparing in advance can make a real difference to your healthy lifestyle and stop you bingeing on 'garbage' when you're hungry.

STOCK UP ON VEGETABLES

Your plate can never be too full of vegetables. Not only are their colours appealing to look at but they pack a mighty nutritional punch too. So, stock up on seasonal vegetables that your skin will love!

READ LABELS

Always read labels so you know exactly what it is that you are eating or putting onto your skin. It's true, 'You are what you eat'.

STAYING HYDRATED IS IMPORTANT... BUT IT'S MORE IMPORTANT TO DO IT THE RIGHT WAY

Drink lots of water and if you like to spice it up a little, I recommend swapping those sugary drinks for water infused with fruit. Or, how about trying one of my favourites from ginger, lemon, mint, orange, or pineapple?

MAKE YOUR OWN HEALTHY SNACKS

Snacking is something many of us do, especially when that sugar craving kicks in. Making your own snacks is not only satisfying to do and gives you a real sense of achievement, but it also means you can fuel your body with healthy nutritious ingredients that your skin will thank you for!

SAVOUR YOUR FOOD

Digestion is key to a healthy gut, which in turn can often show on your skin, so help yours out by getting into the habit of sitting down to eat and taking your time. After all, food is there to be enjoyed.

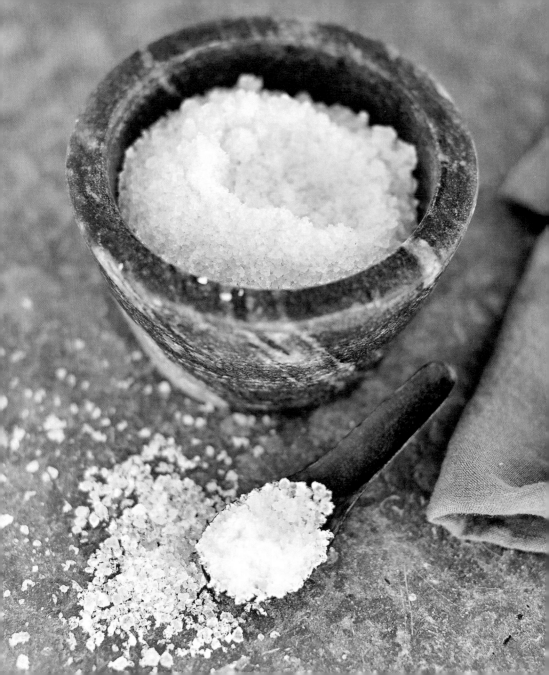

FOR THE BODY

PAMPERING BODY SCRUB

(Makes 1 x 150g or 5½ oz. jar)

Exfoliating the body lifts away dead cells on the skin's surface, leaving skin looking brighter. It also revs up the circulation, helping to drain away trapped water and toxins. The coconut oil and honey in this recipe act as emulsifiers, while the Epsom salts buff the skin's surface and prevent irritation.

> 100g (3½ oz./10 tbsp) Lucy Bee coconut oil
> 2 tbsp honey
> 50g (2 oz./¼ cup) Lucy Bee Epsom salts
> 10 drops favourite essential oil, such as rose geranium + patchouli, lavender + chamomile (optional)

Mash the coconut oil in a medium mixing bowl until it turns soft, then stir in the honey. Add the Epsom salts and essential oil, if using. Stir until smooth, then store in a small glass jar.

TRY THIS! >>>

Step into the shower and, before turning the water on, massage a marble-sized amount of body scrub all over your body (including between your fingers) for 30–60 seconds, avoiding sensitive areas or broken skin. Shower as normal, then pat the skin dry. Repeat 1–2 times per week.

CELLULITE-BUSTING COFFEE BODY SCRUB

(Makes 1 x 150g or 5½ oz. jar)

Those tell-tale dimples on the thighs, bottom, and abdomen happen to the best of us; even models and celebrities aren't immune. Contrary to popular belief, cellulite isn't so much down to fat but your body's septae – a fancy word for the fibrous bands that connect layers of tissue under the skin. Unfortunately, in women they pull at perpendicular angles, causing fat cells to bulge through the bands (think of a fishnet stocking pulled tight over your skin). Other factors, such as age and genes, also play a role. While nothing can completely get rid of cellulite, using a body scrub rich in coffee can at least improve its appearance. Caffeine is one of the best weapons against cellulite as it helps to tighten the skin when applied topically. Here, we combine ground coffee with skin-smoothing coconut oil and a little Himalayan salt to exfoliate and get the lymph and blood moving, so you flush out more trapped fluids.

> 40g (1½ oz./½ cup) organic ground coffee
> 3 tbsp Lucy Bee Himalayan salt
> ½ tbsp Lucy Bee cinnamon powder (optional, for fragrance)
> 100g (3½ oz./10 tbsp) Lucy Bee coconut oil, melted

Combine the coffee, salt and cinnamon, if using, in a mixing bowl. Add the melted coconut oil and mix it in well. Leave to cool before using or transferring to a glass jar.

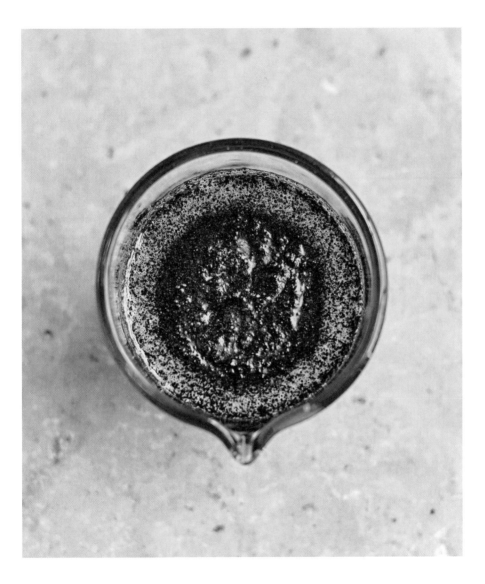

SOOTHING MASSAGE OIL

(Makes enough for 1 application)

The massage oils used in your spa treatment tend to have either coconut or jojoba oil as their base. So next time you fancy a rub down, cut out the middleman and go straight to the bottle. Coconut oil is a great carrier for essential oils.

> 20g (¾ oz./2 tbsp) Lucy Bee coconut oil, melted
> 5–10 drops lavender or rose essential oil

Pour the melted coconut oil into a small mixing bowl. Stir in the lavender or rose essential oil for a soothing massage mix. Apply to skin, transferring any leftovers to a jar.

POST-GYM BODY OIL

(Makes enough for 1 application)

Eucalyptus is an anti-inflammatory, perfect for relieving sore muscles after a rigorous workout. Just slather this oil on damp skin after a shower.

> 20g (¾ oz./2 tbsp) Lucy Bee coconut oil, melted
> 5–10 drops eucalyptus essential oil

Pour the melted coconut oil into a small mixing bowl. Stir in the eucalyptus essential oil for an invigorating massage mix. Apply to skin, transferring any leftovers to a jar.

'YOU'LL BE BORED OF ME SAYING THIS BUT A LITTLE GOES A LONG WAY!'

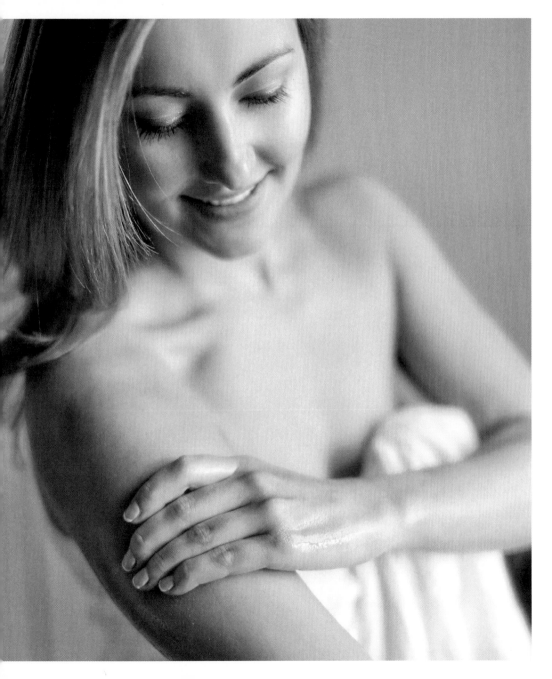

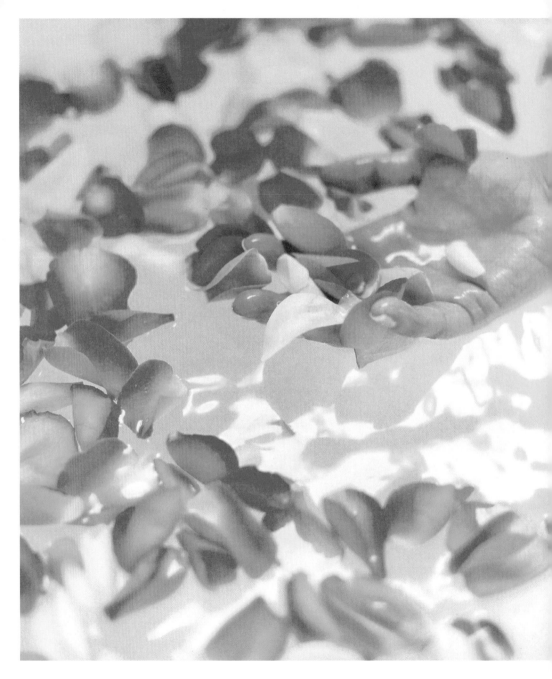

REVITALIZING BATH SOAK

(Makes enough for 1 bath)

Our favourite way to use Lucy Bee Dead Sea salts is in a long, warm bath. With flickering candles and a well-thumbed book, it's the perfect dose of indulgence. Plus the potassium in these salts helps to balance skin moisture, the bromides relax muscles, and magnesium helps you sleep better. Win-win.

> 1 tsp Lucy Bee coconut oil, melted
> 250g (9 oz./1½ cups) Lucy Bee Dead Sea salts
> 10 drops rose or lavender essential oil (optional)
> a few handfuls of fresh rose petals (optional)

After a stressful day, run a warm bath and pour the ingredients into the bath. Lie back and relax for 15–20 minutes to allow the minerals to be absorbed. Be careful when stepping out of the tub, as the bottom may be slippery.

DETOX BATH

(Makes enough for 1 bath)

Many of us are deficient in magnesium. This is partly due to agricultural practices over time, which have affected soil nutrients, but also to poor choices in our diet. What better way to top up on this important mineral than by soaking in a luxurious bath with Epsom salts? Your skin will naturally absorb the magnesium, toxins are drawn out, and tired muscles are relaxed. Lemons have long been known to free up the lymphatic system, the main route for flushing out excess water, and toxins from the body.

> 1 tsp Lucy Bee coconut oil, melted
> 250g (9 oz./1½ cups) Lucy Bee Epsom salts
> 5 drops lemon essential oil
> 5 drops eucalyptus essential oil

After a stressful day, run a warm bath and pour the ingredients into the bath. Lie back and relax for 15–20 minutes to allow the minerals to be absorbed. Be careful when stepping out of the tub, as the bottom may be slippery.

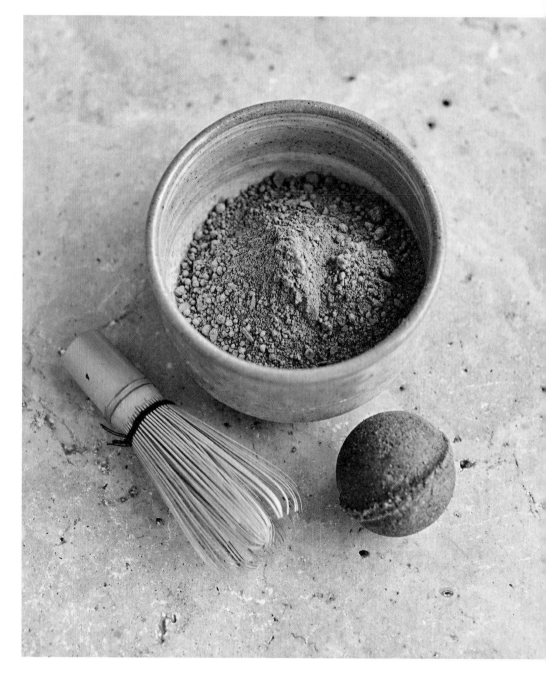

GREEN TEA BATH BOMBS

(Makes 6)

Added to a bath bomb, green tea feeds skin essential nutrients, the coconut oil hydrates, and the lemon oil purifies while also creating an uplifting scent. Take care when handling citric acid on its own and avoid any contact with the skin or eyes while measuring it, as it can cause stinging and irritation. If you really want to splash out you can use matcha green tea powder, which is packed with antioxidants and magnesium-rich chlorophyll (also responsible for its bright green colour).

> 4 tbsp Lucy Bee coconut oil, melted
> 240g (9 oz./1½ cups) bicarbonate of soda (baking soda)
> 120g (4½ oz./¾ cup) citric acid
> 5 tbsp green tea powder
> 5 drops lemon essential oil

Pour the coconut oil into a small mixing bowl. Add the bicarbonate of soda (baking soda) and citric acid (avoiding skin contact with the citric acid). Add the green tea powder to the mixing bowl 1 tablespoon at a time, stirring as you go, then add the lemon essential oil. Leave the mixture to cool, then pour into 6 bath bomb moulds or the moulds of a silicone ice cube tray. Place in the refrigerator for an hour until hard, then remove the bath bombs from the moulds.

HONEY LAVENDER BATH MELT

(Makes 6)

Lavender has been proven to lower stress hormones, slow down heart rate and calm the nervous system. So what better way to use it than in a warm bath after a hectic day? We've included honey and coconut oil to leave your skin feeling silky smooth from top to toe.

> 1 tbsp Lucy Bee coconut oil
> 50g (2 oz./3½ tbsp) shea butter
> 1 tbsp honey
> 10–20 drops lavender essential oil
> 1 tbsp dried lavender buds

Melt the coconut oil and shea butter together (see page 30) until they are a semi-clear liquid. Remove from the heat and pour into a small mixing bowl. Stir in the honey, lavender oil and dried lavender buds. Leave the mixture to cool, then pour into 6 moulds of an ice cube tray. Place in the refrigerator for an hour until hard, then remove the bath melts from the moulds.

'YOU CAN BUY SPECIAL BATH BOMB MOULDS ONLINE – THEY COME IN LOTS OF DIFFERENT SHAPES AND SIZES.'

WHIPPED COCONUT BODY BUTTER

(Makes around 250g or 9 oz.)

If you love the moisturizing benefits of coconut oil but miss the airy, spreadable texture of a regular body butter, try whipping up your coconut oil with a hand mixer.

> 50g (2 oz./5 tbsp) Lucy Bee coconut oil
> 125g (4½ oz./9 tbsp) shea butter
> 50g (2 oz./5 tbsp) olive oil
> 5–10 drops lavender essential oil

Melt the coconut oil and shea butter together (see page 30) with the olive oil added until they turn into a semi-clear liquid. Remove from the heat and refrigerate until the mixture turns white and solid. Then, using a hand mixer, whip up the mixture until it takes on a fluffy texture. Add the lavender oil and continue beating to incorporate. Place inside a glass jar and refrigerate for another hour.

TRY THIS! >>>

If your skin is exceptionally dry, apply the body butter to damp skin, straight after a shower or bath, while the pores are still open. Dermatologists agree that the water droplets on your skin and steam in the bathroom will help the ingredients to penetrate deeper.

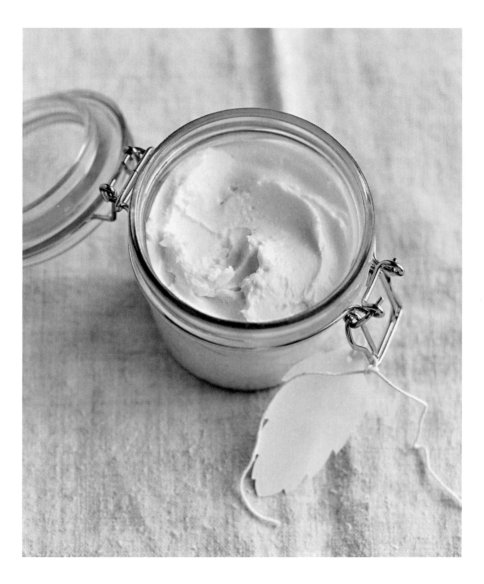

COCONUT OIL SHAVING CREAM

Of all the bathroom essentials, shaving cream is the last thing you should be spending a lot of money on. Coconut oil is an inexpensive, chemical-free alternative.

Use about 15g (½ oz.), melted. Apply a thin layer to the skin and shave straight away. As well as a closer shave, your legs and underarms are left smooth and hydrated.

JUST USE COCONUT OIL!

DEODORANT

Yes, there is such a thing as a natural deodorant that actually works! Spoon out a thimbleful of coconut oil and smooth on your underarms.

JUST USE COCONUT OIL!

AFTERSUN SOOTHER

(Makes 1 x 50g or 2 oz. jar)

The key to treating sunburn is to rehydrate the skin as quickly as possible. This helps assist skin repair and protects against further damage by sealing in moisture.

> 50g (2 oz./5 tbsp) Lucy Bee coconut oil, melted
> 5 drops lavender essential oil

Pour the melted coconut oil into a small mixing bowl and stir in the lavender oil. Leave to cool before applying or transferring to a glass bottle or jar.

'DECANT A SMALL AMOUNT OF COCONUT OIL INTO A MINIATURE TRAVEL POT AND TAKE WITH YOU ON HOLIDAY. IF YOU'RE GOING SOMEWHERE HOT, YOU WON'T EVEN HAVE TO MELT THE OIL!'

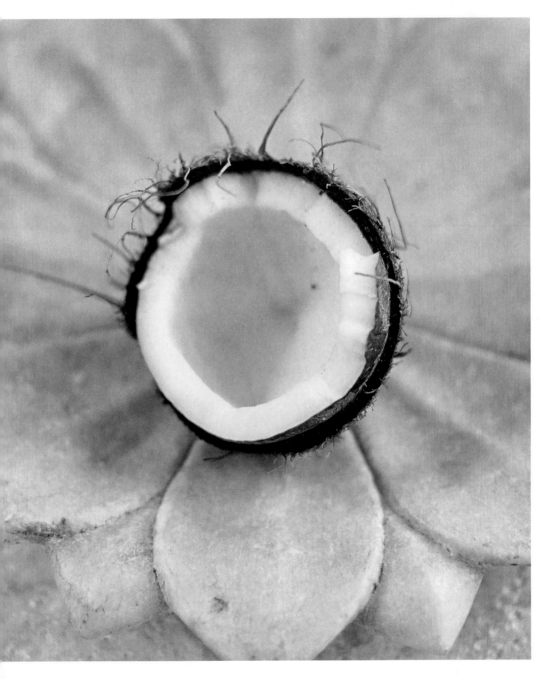

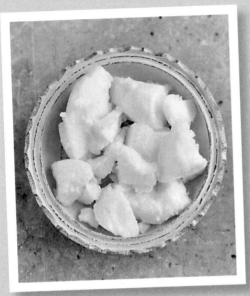

STRETCH MARK CREAM

(Makes enough for 5 applications)

Expectant mums should keep a jar of coconut oil to hand to help ward off stretch marks. Coconut oil is primarily composed of fatty acids, which trap water in the skin to hydrate it – something you'll need as your bump stretches and skin gets drier. Jasmine oil should be avoided during pregnancy as it is a potent aromatherapy oil but post-birth, add a few drops to your coconut oil to turbo-charge its benefits. Jasmine oil is a cicatriser, meaning it helps fade scars left in the wake of stretch marks.

> 2 tbsp Lucy Bee coconut oil
> 2 tbsp shea butter
> 3–4 drops jasmine essential oil (optional)

Melt the coconut oil and shea butter together until they turn into a liquid (see page 30). Remove from the heat and pour into a small mixing bowl. Stir in the jasmine oil, if using, and leave to cool before applying or transferring to a glass bottle or jar.

BABY MASSAGE OIL

(Makes enough for 1 application)

Massage is a lovely way to strengthen the bond between mother and child and helps to relax your baby in time for bed, which is why we've added lavender oil to the blend.

> 10g (⅓ oz./1 tbsp) Lucy Bee coconut oil, melted
> 2 drops lavender essential oil (optional)

Pour the melted coconut oil into a small mixing bowl and stir in the lavender oil, if using. Leave to cool before applying or transferring to a glass bottle or jar. Very gently rub 1 tsp of the mixture into your baby's skin, starting with the legs. For the chest and tummy, gently place both hands flat against the centre of the body and use your fingertips to stroke outwards in small circles.

NAPPY RASH CREAM

Nappy rash can be caused by the nappy rubbing against your baby's skin and even by alcohol-based baby wipes. Treat it with neat coconut oil — being completely raw, organic and natural, this is the best thing for your little one's skin.

Warm 1 tsp of coconut oil between your fingertips and smooth onto the red patches on your baby's bottom.

JUST USE COCONUT OIL!

CRADLE CAP TREATMENT

(Makes enough for 1 application)

Cradle cap is a harmless, non-infectious skin condition in babies and infants, classed as a form of dermatitis that tends to disappear on its own. It appears primarily on the scalp as scaly skin and can have a yellow or brown appearance. Coconut oil can be used as a natural treatment for cradle cap as it is antibacterial and it hydrates the skin. The lauric acid in coconut oil is also antifungal.

Apply 1 tsp of coconut oil to your baby's head and leave on for 20 minutes before rinsing with a mild shampoo. Gently comb the hair to lift away loose flakes.

JUST USE COCONUT OIL!

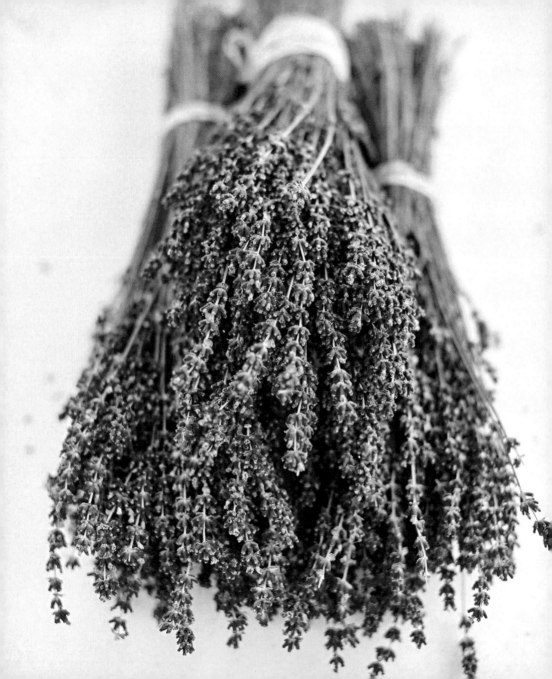

FOR THE HANDS & FEET

CITRUS FOOT SOAK

(Makes enough for 1 use)

Dipping hard-working feet in this foot soak does more than just clean them. The coconut oil softens dead skin cells in preparation for exfoliation, the Epsom salts soothe aching soles, while the lemon oil is antibacterial and antifungal.

> 1 tsp Lucy Bee coconut oil
> 125g (4½ oz./¾ cup) Lucy Bee Epsom salts
> 4 drops lemon essential oil
> 2–3 slices of lemon

Fill a large bowl with lukewarm water. Stir in the coconut oil and, once melted, add the Epsom salts, lemon essential oil and lemon slices. Leave the mixture to soak into your feet for 5–10 minutes then gently pat them dry with a towel.

'TREAT YOUR FEET!'

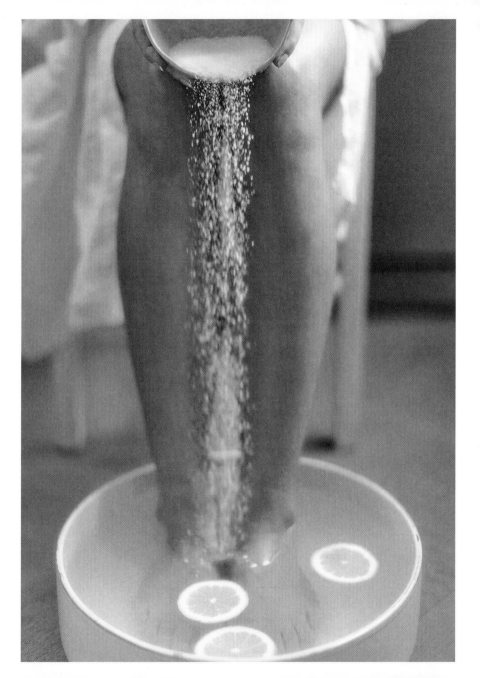

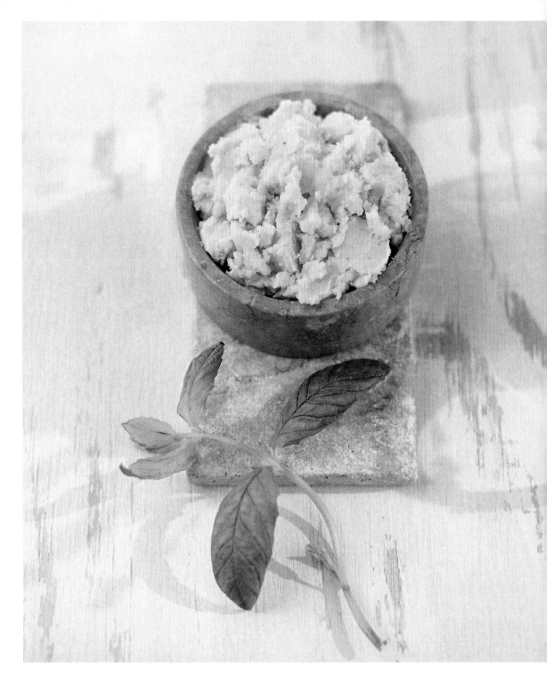

PEPPERMINT FOOT SCRUB

(Makes 375g or 13½ oz.)

Feet still feeling a little rough around the edges? Buff away any calluses and dead skin with this recipe. We promise that your feet have never felt so smooth.

> 250g (9 oz./1½ cups) Lucy Bee coconut oil, melted
> 125g (4½ oz./¾ cup) Lucy Bee Himalayan salt
> 10 drops peppermint essential oil

Pour the melted coconut oil into a small mixing bowl. Add the Himalayan salt and peppermint oil and mix well. Leave to cool before using or transferring to a glass jar, stirring every so often as it cools to avoid separation. Massage each foot for a minute or two with a handful of scrub. Start at your heel and work your way out to your toes, ankles and calves, using tiny circular motions. Rinse off with warm water.

SOOTHING FOOT TREATMENT

(Makes enough for 1 treatment)

After exfoliating your feet, the best thing you can do is drench your soles with a moisturizer made especially for your feet. I've included coconut oil and shea butter to hydrate, lemon to tackle fungal infections, and lavender to reduce inflammation and fragrance your feet.

> 1 tbsp Lucy Bee coconut oil
> 1 tbsp shea butter
> 5 drops lemon essential oil
> 5 drops lavender essential oil

Melt the coconut oil and shea butter together until they turn into a liquid (see page 30). Remove from the heat and pour into a small mixing bowl. Stir in the lemon and lavender essential oils and leave to cool before using or transferring to a glass jar. Generously apply over your feet and use your knuckles to knead into the arch of each foot. Put on a pair of socks to lock in the moisture overnight, or wrap your feet loosely in plastic wrap. Repeat 2–3 times a week until the condition improves and skin feels soft to the touch.

HONEY AND APPLE CIDER VINEGAR CUTICLE CREAM

(Makes enough for 1 week)

It's important to care for your cuticles, as they stimulate new nail growth by increasing circulation in the nail bed. They also protect by sealing off the opening between your nail and the finger itself. You can just massage raw coconut oil into your fingertips but to really turbo-charge its effects, add skin-conditioning raw honey and a splash of apple cider vinegar to balance the skin's pH for healthy nail growth.

> 1 tsp apple cider vinegar
> 1 tsp honey
> 1 tsp Lucy Bee coconut oil, melted

Add the apple cider vinegar and honey to the coconut oil and mix well. Rub over each cuticle, ideally before going to bed when you won't be dipping your hands in and out of water, which causes weakness in the nail.

'TREAT YOUR NAILS AND CUTICLES TO SOME COCONUT OIL WHILE YOU'RE IN THE KITCHEN WAITING FOR DINNER TO COOK!'

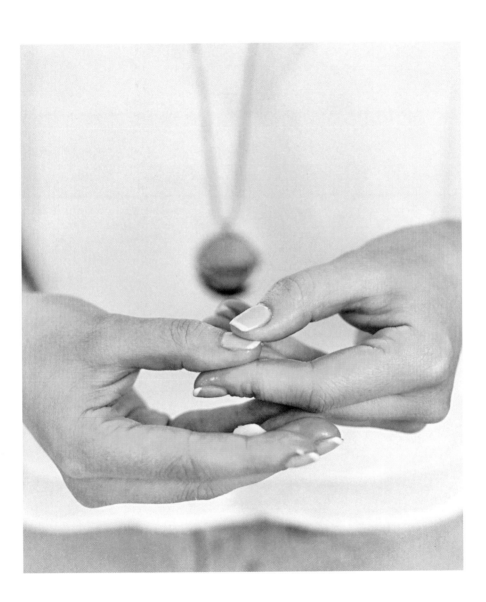

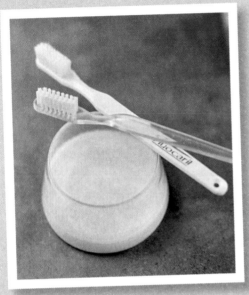

(Makes enough for 1 month)

A bright white smile can make you look healthier and more attractive. But you don't need to fork out hundreds of pounds for a costly tooth whitening treatment at the dentist to erase those caffeine or red wine stains. Simply add bicarbonate of soda (baking soda) to coconut oil for a quick fix. Together they neutralize the bacteria in your mouth that are responsible for destroying tooth enamel.

> 5 tbsp Lucy Bee coconut oil
> 5 tbsp bicarbonate of soda (baking soda)
> 2 drops edible essential oil, such as
>   peppermint or citrus (optional, for flavour)

Simply mix the ingredients together, then transfer to a jar and store at room temperature so it stays solid. Use as you would your regular toothpaste.

OIL PULLING

By practising good oral hygiene (such as flossing, brushing your teeth, and regular trips to the dentist), you'll help to stop the build-up of plaque and tartar, which are the main causes of gum disease and tooth decay. The ancient Ayurvedic practice of oil pulling also plays a key role in maintaining good oral health. The practice is simple: on waking, swish your mouth with coconut oil for 5–20 minutes. Not only does this clean your mouth, but it helps with bloating and sinuses too!

> 1 tsp Lucy Bee coconut oil

Use a teaspoon to scoop out the solid coconut oil and put it into your mouth to melt it. Swirl and swish it around in your mouth like a mouthwash. Push and pull it through your teeth and around your gums. Do this for anywhere between 5 and 20 minutes. Do not swallow the oil – the idea is to get rid of the 'nasties'. Spit it out into a bin as the oil will solidify in your sink and may block it.

JUST USE COCONUT OIL!

'MY TEETH HAVE NEVER FELT SO CLEAN SINCE I STARTED OIL PULLING!'

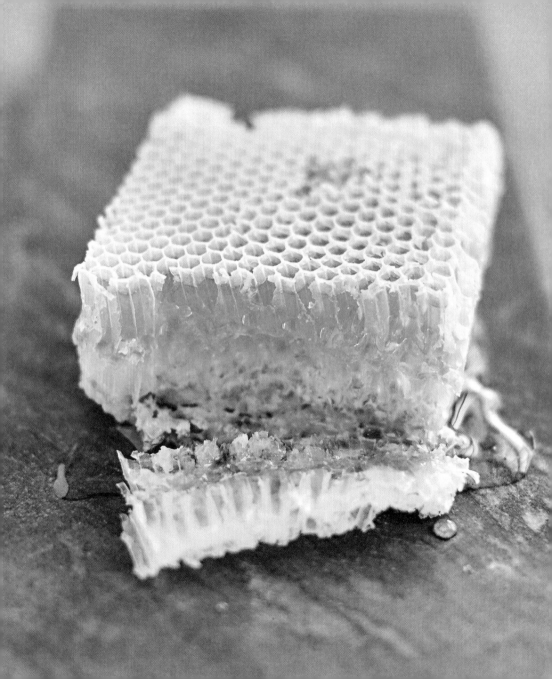

FOR THE HAIR

HONEY AND COCONUT HAIR MASK

*(Makes enough for 1 use
on mid-length hair)*

There's a reason many regular conditioners contain coconut oil: it's able to penetrate hair (and prevent protein loss) better than other oils. It's also loaded with fatty acids that work with the natural proteins found in hair to protect it from breaking and encourage it to grow strong.

> 1 tbsp Lucy Bee coconut oil
> 1 tbsp honey
> 1 tbsp apple cider vinegar (optional, for extra shine)

In a bowl, mash together the coconut oil and honey, with the apple cider vinegar if using, until they form a paste. Apply after shampooing, working the paste through your hair from roots to tips. Leave it on for 2–3 minutes then rinse.

TRY THIS! >>>
Leave in the hair mask as long as possible for the best results.

INTENSIVE COCONUT HAIR MASK

*(Makes enough for 1 use
on mid-length hair)*

Twice a week, use this fortifying blend to repair hair that has been damaged by straighteners or over-processed from bleach.

> 1 tbsp Lucy Bee coconut oil
> 1 tbsp coconut butter
> 5–10 drops essential oil, either chamomile for brightening fair hair, or rosemary for deepening the colour of darker strands

Melt the coconut oil and coconut butter together until they turn into a liquid (see page 30). Remove from the heat and pour into a small mixing bowl. Stir in your chosen essential oil. Leave to cool a little and, while the mixture is still warm, apply a liberal amount to towel-dried hair, concentrating on the mid-lengths to ends where strands tend to be driest and most damaged. Wear a shower cap or wrap your hair in a warm towel as the heat will encourage the nutrients to penetrate deeper into the hair shaft. Leave the mask on for 30 minutes then rinse – or better still, unwrap your hair, spread the towel over your pillow and sleep in the mask.

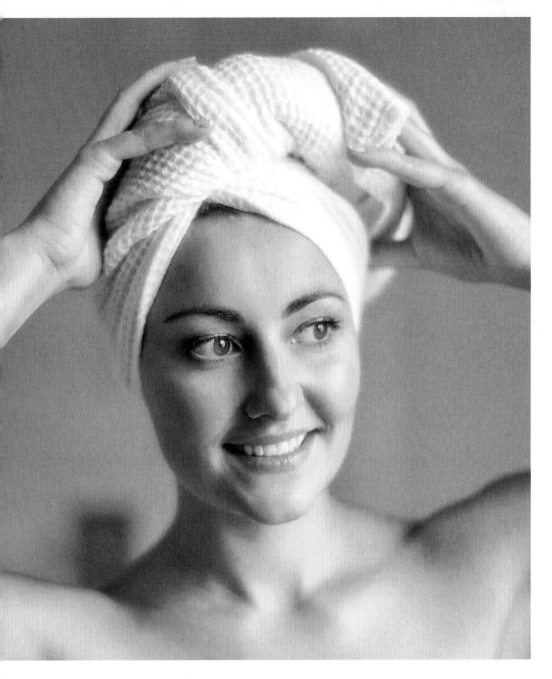

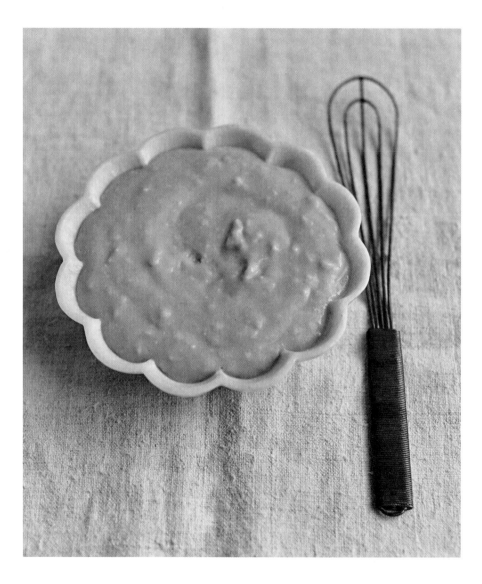

INTENSIVE HAIR MASK FOR COLOURED HAIR

(Makes enough for 1 use on mid-length hair)

For dry, brittle or heat-/colour-damaged hair.

> 2 eggs
> 1 tbsp Lucy Bee coconut oil
> 1 avocado, roughly chopped
> 1 tsp bentonite clay powder

Whisk all the ingredients together. Apply the mixture to your hair in sections. Work into your hair with your fingers, paying special attention to the ends. Cover your hair with a damp, warm towel and leave overnight. Shampoo and condition your hair as usual.

TRY THIS! >>>

Turbo-charge the effects of your hair mask by massaging the paste into your hair with your fingertips, ensuring you really work it into the roots. This helps to boost scalp circulation, meaning more oxygen and nutrients will be sent right to your hair follicles, helping to stimulate growth.

DIY SALT SPRAY

(Makes about 50ml or 2 fl. oz.)

Salt spray adds volume and a beachy texture to even limp, fine strands. Coconut oil prevents the salt from drying out your hair so you can style with confidence.

> 50ml (2 fl. oz./3½ tbsp) hot water (filtered if you live in a hard water area)
> ½ tsp Lucy Bee Epsom salts
> ¼ tsp Lucy Bee coconut oil

Pour the hot water into a 100ml (3½ fl. oz.) spray bottle, then add the Epsom salts and coconut oil. Shake up the mixture and spray liberally onto towel-dried hair, then scrunch the ends until you hair has completely air-dried.

TRY THIS! >>>
When the water in the DIY Salt Spray cools down the coconut oil will solidify. Pop the bottle on top of a heater or radiator for a few minutes to re-melt.

DANDRUFF-BLITZING TREATMENT

(Makes enough for 1 treatment)

Coconut oil and tea tree oil both have antimicrobial and antifungal properties to help control dandruff. And as dandruff and a dry scalp go hand in hand, coconut oil has the added benefit of replacing the scalp's natural oils, thereby restoring the moisture balance.

> 1 tsp Lucy Bee coconut oil, melted
> 3–5 drops tea tree oil

Pour the melted coconut oil into a small mixing bowl. Stir in the tea tree oil and leave to cool a little before using. Massage into the roots and leave it on for 30 minutes – better still overnight – before rinsing. You may need to repeat this process a few times.

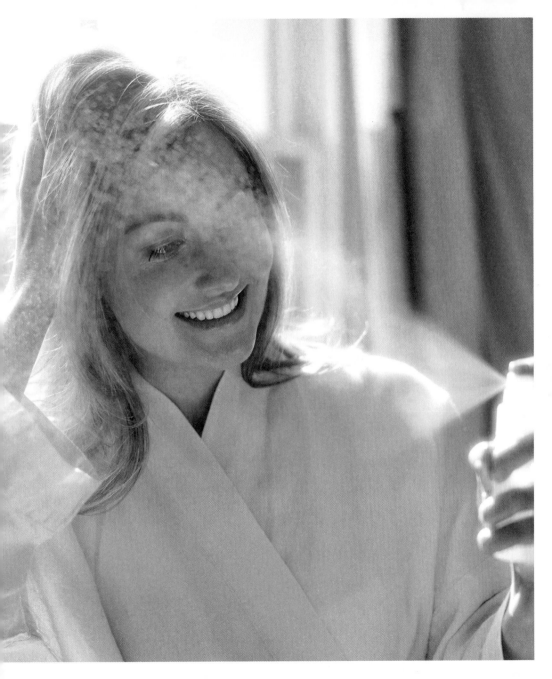

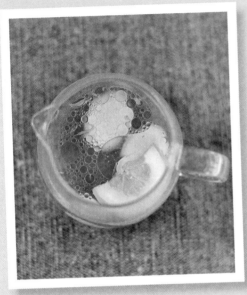

SORE THROAT REMEDY

(Makes enough for 1 use)

This drink is my secret weapon against a cold and scratchy coughs.

> 1 ginger and lemon tea bag
> 1 tsp Lucy Bee coconut oil
> 1 tsp honey

Put the tea bag into a cup and pour boiling water into the cup. Stir in the coconut oil and honey. Sip and enjoy.

'I LOVE USING NATURAL REMEDIES WHERE POSSIBLE TO HEAL MYSELF.'

COCONUT HEALER (FOR CUTS AND RECENT TATTOOS)

(Makes enough for 1 application)

Moisturizing coconut oil can be used as a topical cream for cuts and scrapes — even recent tattoos — to protect against infection while conditioning the skin to heal faster.

Apply 1 tsp of melted coconut oil, or as much as needed, to the wound three times a day. Use until the wound has scabbed over.

SPOT ZAPPER

(Makes enough for about 10 applications)

It might sounds odd to use an oil on oily skin but the antimicrobial properties of coconut make it an ideal natural choice.

> 1 tsp Lucy Bee coconut oil, melted
> 2 drops tea tree essential oil

Pour the melted coconut oil into a small mixing bowl and add the tea tree oil. Leave to cool before using, or pouring into a glass container. Store in the refrigerator so the mixture solidifies and the cold temperature reduces inflammation. Use a cotton bud to apply directly to the spot as needed.

DIY MOSQUITO SPRAY

(Makes about 50ml or 2 fl. oz.)

Ease the itching from mosquito bites by applying this blend onto affected areas. Tea tree oil is antiseptic and the magnesium-rich Epsom salts kick-start the body's healing mechanisms.

> 50ml (2 fl. oz./3½ tbsp) hot water (filtered if you live in a hard water area)
> 2 tbsp Lucy Bee Epsom salts
> 5 drops tea tree oil

Pour the hot water into a 100ml (3½ fl. oz.) spray bottle then add the Epsom salts and tea tree oil. Shake up the mixture. Either mist directly onto bites or spray onto a cotton wool ball and apply.

INDEX

THANK YOUS

My first thank you is to my **mum, Natalie and dad, Phil,** for always being so supportive in everything I choose to do. It's the best feeling knowing I am working alongside my family and that so many exciting things are happening. Love you both.
David Loftus – What an incredible experience it has been working alongside you on this book. Who knew yogurt could look so good?! Thank you so much for everything, I love it! **Maria Comparetto** – Thank you for my flawless make-up, it looked stunning. I didn't want to take it off (with my coconut oil, obviously) even at the end of the day.
Poppy Mahon – It was great working with you again, you are now a pro at making green tea bath bombs, you are so talented and a great laugh to be around. Thank you.
Helen Lewis – It was really good working with you on this book and thanks for your organisation and gluten-free lunches, I had so much fun. **Katherine Keeble** – Another beautifully styled book, thanks for bringing your creativity to the project. **Lisa Pendreigh** – Thank you for making both books happen; food and beauty – two of my favourite things. Thanks for sharing all your great ideas with us! **Amy Christian** – Thank you for all your hard work in making sure the book is perfect, I've really appreciated it. **Fiona Embleton** – Thank you so much for all your help and research for this book. It's been great working with you and I loved our chats on all things beauty. **Petrina Grint** – Thank you so much for being there 24/7. Whenever I need any help you are the first one to call. It was great being at the shoot with you.
Hannah Grint – Thank you for all the laughs and help throughout the process of both books. Finally, a huge thank you to our followers, who continue to inspire me every day.

 Lucy Bee x